Mediterranean Diet for Beginners

The Complete Guide to Get Started Delicious and Healthy Mediterranean Diet Recipes to Lose Weight, Gain Energy and Fat Burn.

Disclaimer

The Mediterranean Diet has been rated as one of the most beneficial diets for human health, beating the Keto diet, Atkins diet, and even the vegetarian diet.

Rich in healthy, fresh produce and without calorie restriction, carb control or any similar kind of restriction, it's an incredible way to lose weight, rebalance your body and live longer.

That's why I've written this book- to show you how you can enjoy the wide variety of delicious foods, look and feel at your best and enjoy many mouth-watering, easy and inexpensive recipes along the way.

Having said that, remember that I'm not a medical professional and I'm not qualified to give you medical advice. For that reason, please consult a medical professional before taking part in this diet, especially if you have a pre-existing health problem. By following this diet, you agree to do so at your own risk and assume all associated risk involved.

The information in this book is for informational purposes only and is not intended to be construed as medical advice nor should it replace the guidance of a qualified instructor who can guide you personally and tailor the Mediterranean diet to your specific needs and requirements.

Bear in mind that there are no 'typical' results from the information provided - as individuals differ, the results will differ.

No responsibility is taken for any loss or damage related directly or indirectly to the information in this book. Never disregard professional medical advice or delay in seeking it because of something you have read in this book or in any linked materials.

Copyright © 2019 xx

All rights reserved. No part of this publication may be reproduced, distributed, or transmitted in any form or by any means, including photocopying, recording, or other electronic or mechanical methods, without the prior written permission of the publisher.

Table of Contents

Introduction — 7
- What is the Mediterranean diet? — 7
- What are the benefits of the Mediterranean diet? — 7
- What should you eat on the Mediterranean diet? — 8
- What foods should you avoid on the Mediterranean diet? — 9
- What you can drink — 9
- What about snacks? — 9
- How to eat out when you're following the Mediterranean diet? — 10

Recipes — 11
- Breakfasts — 11
  - Egg Caprese Breakfast Cups — 11
  - Honey Almond Ricotta Spread with Peaches — 12
  - Caprese Avocado Toast — 13
  - Feta & Quinoa Egg Muffins — 14
  - Greek Yogurt Pancakes — 15
  - Asparagus and Mushroom Frittata with Goat Cheese — 16
  - Mediterranean Egg Bake Strata — 17
  - Mini Breakfast Frittata — 18
- Salads — 19
  - Greek Chicken Gyro Salad — 19
  - Tuscan Tuna and White Bean Salad — 20
  - Avocado Caprese Salad — 21
  - Quinoa and Kale Protein Power Salad — 22
  - Greek Pasta Salad with Cucumbers & Artichoke Hearts — 23
  - Arugula Salad with Pesto Shrimp, Parmesan and Beans — 24
  - Autumn Couscous — 25
  - Greek Salad with Avocado — 26
  - Garlicky Swiss Chard and Garbanzo Beans — 27
  - Citrus Shrimp and Avocado Salad — 28
  - Mediterranean-Style Mustard Potato Salad — 29
  - Herby Tuna Salad with Lime Dressing — 30
- Soups — 31
  - White Bean Soup — 31

- Roasted Red Pepper and Tomato Soup --- 32
- Moroccan Lentil Soup --- 33
- Greek Lemon Chicken Soup --- 34
- Minestrone Soup --- 35
- Simple Zucchini & Garlic Soup --- 36
- Chicken Leek Soup with White Wine --- 37
- Italian Meatball Soup --- 38
- Greek Easter Lamb Soup --- 40
- Tuscan White Bean Soup with Sausage and Kale --- 41

Sandwiches & Wraps --- 42
- Mediterranean Tuna Sandwiches --- 42
- Avocado Feta Wrap --- 43
- Pesto Goat Cheese Eggplant Wrap --- 43
- Mediterranean Hummus Wrap --- 44
- Mediterranean Chicken Wraps with Hummus --- 45
- Easy Chicken Sandwiches --- 46
- Falafel Pitta Sandwich --- 47
- Mediterranean Veggie Sandwich with Smoked Tofu --- 48
- Hummus and Vegetable Sandwich --- 49
- Mediterranean Black Olive Hummus Paninis --- 50
- Mediterranean Turkey Panini --- 51
- Italian Panini Grill Sandwich --- 52
- Avocado Caprese Wrap --- 53

Chicken & Turkey --- 54
- Grilled Balsamic Chicken with Olive Tapenade --- 54
- Greek Chicken Marinade --- 56
- Chicken Quinoa Bowl with Broccoli & Tomato --- 57
- Greek Chicken Kebab --- 58
- Quick Caprese Chicken --- 59
- Grilled Greek Lemon Chicken Skewers --- 60
- Greek Turkey Burgers with Tzatziki Sauce --- 61
- One-Skillet Tomato and Olive Chicken --- 62
- Chicken Pasta Bake --- 63
- Mozzarella Chicken Bake --- 65

- Spiced Mediterranean Chicken — 66
- One Pot Greek Chicken & Lemon Rice — 67
- Harissa Chicken with Garbanzo Beans and Sweet Potatoes — 69

Seafood — 70
- Linguine and Zucchini Noodles with Shrimp — 70
- Shrimp Pasta with Roasted Red Peppers and Artichokes — 71
- Baked Shrimp and Veggies — 72
- Easy Baked Octopus — 73
- Saucy Greek Baked Shrimp — 74
- Italian Seafood Stew — 75

Fish — 76
- Baked Fish with Artichokes and Olives — 76
- Salmon with Paprika and Fennel — 77
- Striped Bass with Provencal Tomatoes — 78
- Tuna Couscous with Pepperoncini — 79
- Parmesan Pesto Tilapia — 80
- Rosemary Citrus One Pan Baked Salmon — 81
- Pan-Fried Cod with Orange and Swiss Chard — 82
- Pan-Seared Cod with Pomegranate Salsa — 83
- Honey-Mustard Sheet Pan Salmon — 84
- Fish Puttanesca en Papillote — 85
- Hemp and Walnut Crusted Salmon with Broccoli and Kimchi Cauliflower Rice — 86
- Spiced Moroccan Halibut — 87
- Sicilian Style Salmon with Garlic Broccoli and Tomatoes — 88
- Sardines with Fennel and Orange — 89
- Sardine and Chili Fettuccine with Pine Nuts and Lemon — 90

Vegetarian & Vegan — 91
- Vegan Moussaka — 91
- Stuffed Grape Leaves Casserole — 93
- Paella Primavera — 94
- Portuguese Tomato Rice — 95

Appetizers and Side Dishes — 96
- Greek Spinach and Rice — 96
- Greek Style Green Beans — 97

- Roasted Potatoes with Lemon and Garlic — 98
- Herb Roasted Olives — 99
- Peach Bruschetta — 100
- Goat Cheese Mushrooms — 101
- Mediterranean Crab Phyllo Cups — 102

Dips & Spreads — 103
- Greek Eggplant Dip — 103
- Greek Parsley-Garlic Dip — 104
- Easy Ful Medammes — 105
- Red Pepper Dip with Feta Cheese and Greek Yogurt — 106
- Tzatziki — 107

Desserts & Sweet Treats — 108
- Greek Yogurt Chocolate Mousse — 108
- Pistachio Mascarpone Cake with Roasted Figs — 109
- Vegan Coffee Tiramisu — 111
- Mediterranean Pistachio No Bake Snack Bars — 113

Final words — 114

Introduction

I tried for *such* a long time to find the perfect introduction to this book.

Would I start by telling you that the Mediterranean diet will help you eat all the foods you love, enjoy regular-sized portions of food and still lose weight?

Should I point out that there's an ever-increasing number of people have reached their ideal weight, shed fat and started to live life to the maximum thanks to this incredible diet?

Or would it be better just to tell you that the Mediterranean diet will give you a huge array of the most amazing, mouth-watering, sunshine-filled, uplifting recipes that you could ever taste?

That these foods are packed full of all the vitamins, minerals, antioxidants and phytonutrients that you need to thrive?

The truth is, I just don't know. Because the Mediterranean diet is all these things and much much more.

What is the Mediterranean diet?

According to researchers, the Mediterranean diet is the healthiest diet in the world.

Unlike many other strict diet plans, it emphasizes filling your plate with an abundance of plant-based foods such as vegetables, fruits, wholegrains, legumes, olive oil, fish, seafood, chicken and turkey.

Dairy is consumed regularly but in moderate amounts, red meat and pork are usually omitted or consumed less (if at all) and you can even enjoy a glass or two of red wine in moderation if you fancy.

This is an eating plan that isn't set in stone- you can adjust it according to your personal likes and dislikes and still lose weight and feel great.

Because it's comprised of real foods which have been minimally processed and don't contain additives, preservatives, high-fructose corn syrup, trans fats or any of those potentially harmful ingredients, this diet provides your body with everything you need to look and feel amazing, to effortless shift weight without counting calories, to feel energized and to stay healthier for longer.

What are the benefits of the Mediterranean diet?

As I mentioned earlier, the Mediterranean diet offers a wealth of health benefits. Here are some of the best:

- Helps you to <u>lose weight</u> without feeling deprived

- Gives you <u>more energy</u> and greater athletic performance
- Improves issues with <u>your digestive health</u>
- Boosts <u>brain health</u> and encourages focus and productivity
- Reduces <u>your risk of cancer</u>
- Reduces risk of <u>heart disease</u>
- Lowers risk of <u>Parkinson's and Alzheimer's</u> disease
- Reduces risk of <u>strokes</u> and high blood pressure
- Relieves <u>depression and anxiety</u>
- Helps <u>regulate your blood sugar levels</u> and ease type 2 diabetes and metabolic syndrome
- Helps <u>increase your lifespan</u>

And did I mention that it also gives your taste buds a real treat?

What should you eat on the Mediterranean diet?

You're free to eat a wide range of foods on the Mediterranean Diet provided that they are wholefoods and based on a single ingredient. Think simple, wholesome and vitamin rich. Fill your plate with as many plants as possible and eat fish and seafood at least twice per week.

Exactly which foods belong to the diet is a matter for debate, however, because there is a difference between the culinary habits of the countries around the Mediterranean. Choose whichever foods you love the most.

This might include:

- **Fresh vegetables:** Enjoy a wide range of fresh veggies including tomatoes, broccoli, peppers, kale, spinach, onions, garlic, carrots, cucumber, fennel, zucchini, eggplant and so on. Aim to fill most of your plate with veggies.
- **Fresh fruits:** You can tuck into whatever fruits take your fancy. Why not include apples, bananas, oranges, pears, strawberries, peaches, melons, dates, grapes, figs, blueberries and many of the other options out there?
- **Nuts and seeds:** Enjoy almonds, brazil nuts walnuts, macadamia nuts, hazelnuts, cashews, sunflower seeds, pumpkin seeds, chia seeds, sesame seeds and more.
- **Beans and legumes:** These provide a myriad of health benefits, taste great and even help reduce your food budget. Enjoy all beans, peas, lentils, pulses, peanuts, chickpeas, and so on.
- **Root veggies and tubers:** Yes, you can enjoy potatoes, sweet potatoes, turnips, swede and yams.
- **Wholegrains:** Fill up with whole oats, brown rice, rye, barley, corn, buckwheat, whole wheat, whole-grain bread and pasta.
- **Fish and seafood**: Include salmon, sardines, trout, tuna, mackerel, shrimp, oysters, clams, crab, mussels, and whatever other fish or seafood you fancy.
- **Poultry:** Chicken, duck, turkey is great.
- **Eggs & dairy:** Enjoy fresh eggs, cheese, yoghurt and Greek yoghurt.

- **Fats:** Use extra virgin olive oil, avocados, olives, avocado oil plus nuts and seeds.
- **Herbs and spices:** Get creative and use whatever herbs and spices your heart desires as long as they're not blends which contain additives, preservatives, sugars or sweeteners. We love rosemary, oregano, basil, mint, sage, nutmeg, cinnamon, and cumin for their authentic Mediterranean flavor.

What foods should you avoid on the Mediterranean diet?

You should avoid or reduce your consumption of the following foods:

- **Processed sugars:** Soda, ice cream, candy, chocolate, cakes, cookies and similar.
- **Processed and highly refined grains:** White bread, white pasta and white rice.
- **Refined oils and trans fats:** Margarine, soybean oil, canola oil, cottonseed oil and processed foods which contain these oils.
- **Processed foods:** Processed foods, especially those labelled 'diet' or 'low fat'.
- **Processed meat:** Processed sausages, hot dogs, processed meats, etc.

If you do choose to eat a small amount of processed foods, it's a good idea read the labels carefully to ensure that you're avoiding these unhealthy ingredients. If you can, stick to wholefoods so you can have complete peace of mind that you're doing the best for your body.

What you can drink

Soda, cordials and other processed drinks are off the menu on the Mediterranean diet as they are often full of additives, sugars and other unhealthy ingredients.

Instead stick to water, perhaps flavored with a slice of fresh lemon or lime if preferred.

You can also enjoy unsweetened tea and coffee freely and include small amounts of wine with your evening meal. However, this should be avoided if you have issues with alcohol.

What about snacks?

Most Mediterranean countries don't have a snack culture like we do in the US and stick to eating well-balanced, plant-based meals instead. However, if you're hungry and in need of a snack, you can choose from one of the following:

- Nuts
- Fresh fruit
- Sliced carrots, cucumber and red peppers
- Greek yoghurt
- Apple slices with almond butter
- Leftover food in your fridge

How to eat out when you're following the Mediterranean diet?

Despite what you might think, it's very simple to eat out at most restaurants on this diet. Here's how do it stress-free:

1. Avoid fast-food restaurants and places that sell highly processed junk foods
2. Choose fish, seafood or a healthy vegetarian/vegan dish as your main meal
3. Include plenty of steamed vegetables with your order (ask for extra if needed)
4. Ask them to fry your food in olive oil
5. Opt. for wholegrain bread with olive oil instead of white bread with butter.
6. Enjoy a glass of wine if you want to.
7. If you really want a desert, choose fresh fruit and nuts where available
8. Finish with a freshly brewed coffee or tea if desired (but don't add any sugar!)

As you can see, the Mediterranean diet really is incredible. It allows you to enjoy a wide range of healthy real foods, helps you to lose weight and leaves you looking amazing. What's not to like about it??

So, by now you should be feeling clued up about this diet and ready to dive straight to the recipes, so let's get to it! I've included a range of delicious breakfasts, warming soups, delicious sandwiches and salads, fish and seafood dishes, balanced vegetarian and vegan dishes, tasty side dishes and starters, dips and spreads and even a handful of desert recipes to help you spoil yourself a little.

Remember that there's nothing strict about this diet so feel free to get creative and tweak the recipes until they're exactly to your liking.

Enjoy!

Recipes

Breakfasts

Egg Caprese Breakfast Cups

If you're looking for a simple and fast healthy breakfast that is packed full of flavor and will help kick-start your day the right way, look no further than these Italian-style egg cups. They're delicious, ready quickly and you can throw whatever ingredients in that you like.

Serves: 2
Time: 15 mins
- Calories: 356
- Net carbs: 8g
- Protein: 30g
- Fat: 28g

Ingredients:
- 2 slices thinly sliced ham
- 4 oz. shredded mozzarella
- 2 free-range eggs
- Pesto sauce, to taste
- Cherry tomatoes, halved
- Salt and pepper, to taste

To serve...
- Fresh basil leaves

Method:
1. Find a ramekin or small bowl and brush lightly with oil to prevent sticking.
2. Add the slices of ham to the bottom and up the side, and push into the sides.
3. Sprinkle the cheese over the ham.
4. Crack the eggs into a bowl and pour into the ramekin.
5. Top with a dollop of pesto, a few cherry halves and season to taste.
6. Place into the microwave, cover and cook on high for 1 minute 30 seconds until cooked.
7. Serve with extra basil leaves and enjoy!

Honey Almond Ricotta Spread with Peaches

Enjoy your breakfast with a taste of the Mediterranean when you create this rich, creamy and indulgent-feeling ricotta spread. Surprisingly healthy, it blends the fragrant flavor of fresh peach with honey, almonds and ricotta to make a breakfast spread that beats jelly any day!

Serves: 4-6
Time: 15 mins

- Calories: 347
- Net carbs: 24g
- Protein: 22g
- Fat: 16g

Ingredients:

For the ricotta spread...

- 1 cup whole milk ricotta
- 1/2 cup sliced almonds
- 1/4 teaspoon almond extract
- 1 teaspoons honey
- Zest from an orange, optional

To serve...

- Whole grain toast
- Sliced peaches
- Sliced almonds
- Extra honey, for drizzling

Method:

1. Grab a medium bowl and add the ricotta, almonds and almond extra. Stir well to combine.
2. Sprinkle your optional toppings, including the sliced almonds, honey, peaches and honey.
3. Serve with toast and enjoy!

Caprese Avocado Toast

There are a million different ways you can get your avocado toast fix, but nothing beats the fresh flavors of cottage cheese, tomato, basil and soft and delicious avocado. Tip: freshly ground pepper is the metaphorical icing on the cake with this breakfast. This recipe only serves one, so feel free to double or triple if you have more mouths to feed.

Serves: 1
Time: 5 mins
- Calories: 372
- Net carbs: 37g
- Protein: 15g
- Fat: 21g

Ingredients:
- 1 slice wholewheat toast
- 1-2 teaspoons olive oil
- 1/2 avocado, sliced
- 1/3 cup low-fat cottage cheese
- 1 small tomato, sliced

To serve...
- Basil leaves
- Salt and pepper, to taste

Method:
1. Place your piece of toast onto a plate and drizzle well with olive oil.
2. Add the cottage cheese, the avocado slices and the tomato.
3. Season well with salt and pepper and serve with the basil leaves.
4. Enjoy!

Feta & Quinoa Egg Muffins

These nutrient-packed breakfast muffins combine a wide range of flavors from the Med and bring them all together in a grab-and-go package that will keep you fueled for the whole morning. Enjoy.

Makes: 12
Time: 45 mins

- Calories: 113
- Net carbs: 5g
- Protein: 6g
- Fat: 7g

Ingredients:

- 2 cups baby spinach, finely chopped
- 1/2 cup finely chopped onion
- 1 cup sliced tomatoes
- 1/2 cup chopped Kalamata olives
- 1 tablespoon chopped fresh oregano
- 2 teaspoons olive oil, plus extra for greasing
- 8 free-range eggs
- 1 cup cooked quinoa
- 1 cup crumbled feta cheese
- 1/4 teaspoon salt

Method:

1. Preheat your oven to 350°F, grease a 12-cup baking tin then pop to one side.
2. Pop a skillet over a medium heat and add the oil.
3. Cook the onions for five minutes until soft, then throw in the tomatoes and spinach and cook for a further minute or so.
4. Remove from the heat and stir through the oregano and olives.
5. Break the eggs into a small mixing bowl and whisk well.
6. Add the quinoa, feta, veggies and salt and stir well until mixed through.
7. Pour into the pre-prepared tin and pop into the oven for 30 minutes.
8. Remove from the oven and leave to rest for five minutes.
9. Serve and enjoy!

Greek Yogurt Pancakes

I don't ever want to hear that you've used an instant pancake mix again! This recipe is so easy- just throw everything into a bowl, stir and you're almost done. For best results, make sure your pan is really hot before you start cooking. Yum!

Serves: 6
Time: 30 mins
- Calories: 258
- Net carbs: 32g
- Protein: 11g
- Fat: 8g

Ingredients:
- 1 1/4 cup all-purpose flour
- 1/4 teaspoon salt
- 2 teaspoons baking powder
- 1 teaspoon baking soda
- 1/4 cup sugar
- 3 tablespoons butter unsalted, melted
- 3 free-range eggs
- 1 1/2 cups plain Greek yogurt plain
- 1/2 cup milk
- 1/2 cup blueberries, (opt)

Method:
1. Grab a large bowl and add the flour, salt, baking powder and baking soda. Stir well to combine.
2. Take another bowl and add the sugar, butter, eggs, yoghurt and milk and blend until smooth.
3. Make a small well in the dry ingredients and add the wet ingredients. Stir well until combined.
4. Place a skillet or griddle over a high heat and grease with olive oil or butter.
5. Once smoking hot, add small spoons of the pancake batter and leave until cooked. Flip and cook on the opposite side.
6. Remove and place onto a plate to keep warm.
7. Repeat with the remaining pancake batter and then serve and enjoy.

Asparagus and Mushroom Frittata with Goat Cheese

This frittata is so special that it's a shame just to eat it on the weekends for your brunch. It's fast, it's easy and it's utterly amazing so I highly recommend you make the effort and enjoy it on your weekday mornings too. Any leftovers are also tasty if you can't eat it all at once.

Serves: 1
Time: 30 mins
- Calories: 328
- Net carbs: 4g
- Protein: 18g
- Fat: 26g

Ingredients:
- 2 free-range eggs
- 1 teaspoon water or milk
- Pinch of salt
- Olive oil
- 2-3 brown mushrooms, sliced
- 4-5 asparagus spears, trimmed and cut into ½" pieces
- 1 tablespoon chopped green onion
- 2 tablespoons goat cheese

Method:
1. Preheat your broiler and grease a 7" frying pan with oil.
2. Place the pan over a medium heat then add the mushrooms and cook for five minutes until soft.
3. Add the asparagus and cook for a minute or two more.
4. Break the eggs into a small bowl, add the water and a pinch of salt and whisk well.
5. Pour the eggs over the mushrooms and asparagus, add the onion and goat's cheese and leave to set.
6. Once the egg starts to pull away from the pan, place under the broiler and cook for five minutes until the top browns.
7. Sprinkle with extra goat's cheese then serve and enjoy.

Mediterranean Egg Bake Strata

This incredible egg bake does contain a range of ingredients and takes a little while to cook. That's why it's best to enjoy as a brunch or a holiday treat. If you're into meal planning, you can also make it in advance and reheat throughout the week. Enjoy!

Serves: 4-6
Time: 1 hour 10 mins
- Calories: 365
- Net carbs: 25g
- Protein: 16g
- Fat: 22g

Ingredients:
- 3 tablespoons olive oil
- 2 cloves garlic, minced
- 2 shallots, minced
- 1 cup button mushrooms, sliced
- 1 teaspoon dried marjoram leaves
- 6 cups white bread, cut into ½" chunks
- 1/2 cup artichoke hearts, cut into 1/8s
- 1/4 cup Kalamata olives, quartered
- 1/4 cup marinated sundried tomatoes slivered
- 1/4 cup shredded parmesan cheese plus extra for topping
- 4 oz. mozzarella cheese, halved
- 6 free-range eggs
- 1 1/2 cups half and half
- 1/4 cup basil leaves, slivered
- Salt, to taste

Method:
1. Preheat the oven to 325°F and grease a large baking dish.
2. Place a skillet over a medium heat, add the oil and heat.
3. Add the shallot and garlic and cook for 1-2 minutes until fragrant.
4. Add the mushrooms and marjoram and cook for 5 minutes.
5. Remove from the heat and transfer to a large bowl.
6. Throw in the bread chunks, artichokes, olives, sundried tomatoes and cheeses. Season well.
7. Pour the mixture into the baking dish.
8. Find another bowl and add the eggs, whisking well. Add the half and half and stir well to combine.
9. Pour over the bread mixture then top with more parmesan and basil.
10. Pop into the oven for 50 minutes until the eggs have set.
11. Leave to rest for five minutes, then serve and enjoy!

Mini Breakfast Frittata

Olives, peppers, sundried tomatoes, cheese...my mouth is watering just at the very thought of it! Easy to create and easier still to throw into your bag and enjoy when you're on the run, they're a great taste of the Mediterranean that will nourish you from the inside out!

Serves: 3-6
Time: 20 mins
- Calories: 167
- Net carbs: 6g
- Protein: 9g
- Fat: 12g

Ingredients:
- 6 free-range eggs
- 1/4 cup milk or half and half
- Salt and pepper, to taste
- ¼ cup artichokes in oil, drained and thinly sliced
- ⅓ cup pitted kalamata olives, drained and quartered
- ¼ cup bottled sweet red peppers, drained and chopped
- ½ cup sun-dried tomatoes in oil, drained and chopped
- ¼ cup mozzarella cheese, shredded
- ¼ cup feta cheese, crumbled
- ¼ cup Italian flat leaf parsley, chopped

Method:
1. Preheat your oven to 375°F and grease two mini muffin tins. Pop to one side.
2. Take a medium bowl and add the eggs and milk or half and half. Whisk well to combine.
3. Divide the mixture between the muffin tins, filling to about ¾ full.
4. Divide the remaining ingredients between the pans, dropping into the egg mixture and pushing down if required.
5. Pop into the oven and cook for 10-15 minutes until set and golden.
6. Serve and enjoy.

Salads

Greek Chicken Gyro Salad

This delicious chicken salad is likely to become your go-to salad recipe! Combining the perfect range of textures, taste and crunch, it will be ready quickly and in your stomach fast.

Serves: 2
Time: 15 mins
- Calories: 885
- Net carbs: 82g
- Protein: 46g
- Fat: 48g

Ingredients:
- 6 cups chopped romaine lettuce
- 1 x 8 oz. Greek marinated chicken breast, sliced or chopped
- 1 x 15 oz. can garbanzo beans, drained
- 1 cup cherry tomatoes, sliced
- 1 cup sliced cucumber
- 1/2 avocado, chopped
- 1/4 cup sliced Kalamata olives
- 1/4 cup sliced red onion

For the pitta crisps...
- 2 pitta bread pockets, chopped into triangles
- Olive oil, to taste
- Paprika, to taste
- Tzatziki (recipe available in Dips & Spreads in this book)

For the dressing...
- 1/4 cup extra virgin olive oil
- 1/4 cup red wine vinegar
- 1 clove garlic, peeled and minced
- 2 teaspoons oregano
- 1 teaspoon sugar
- Salt and pepper, to taste

Method:
1. Take a large serving bowl and add the lettuce.
2. Throw in the chicken, garbanzo beans, tomatoes, cucumber, avocado, olives and red onion. Toss well then pop to one side.
3. Take the pitta bread triangles, brush with olive oil, sprinkle with paprika and toast until golden. Pop to one side.
4. Take a small bowl and add the olive oil, vinegar, garlic, oregano, sugar, salt and pepper. Stir well to combine.
5. Pour over the salad and toss to dress.
6. Add the tzatziki and the pitta chips then serve and enjoy!

Tuscan Tuna and White Bean Salad

You can still enjoy an amazing tuna salad without ever needing a drop of mayo! Using a versatile blend of olive oil and lemon juice, you can dress your salad to perfection and take care of your body to the max.

Serves: 2
Time: 15 mins

- Calories: 533
- Net carbs: 42g
- Protein: 29g
- Fat: 32g

Ingredients:

- 4 cups arugula or spinach
- 1 x 15 oz. can cannellini beans, rinsed and drained
- 1 x 5 oz. can white albacore tuna, packed in water drained
- 1/2 cup cherry tomatoes, halved
- 1/4 cup sliced Kalamata olives
- 1 red onion, sliced
- 2 tablespoons extra virgin olive oil
- 1/2 lemon
- 1/4 cup crumbled feta cheese
- Salt and pepper, to taste

Method:

1. Grab a large bowl and add the greens, beans, tuna, tomatoes, olives and red onion. Toss to combine.
2. Add the olive oil and lemon juice and toss again.
3. Top with the feta cheese, season to taste and serve and enjoy.

Avocado Caprese Salad

Give this traditional Italian salad a facelift by adding the nourishing taste of fresh avocado. It's still beautifully simple and will whisk your taste buds away to an island in the sun. Delicious!

Serves: 1-2
Time: 15 mins
- Calories: 591
- Net carbs: 33g
- Protein: 27g
- Fat: 44g

Ingredients:
- 2 cups fresh arugula
- 2-3 cherry tomatoes sliced
- 1/2 avocado, pitted and sliced
- 3 slices fresh mozzarella cheese
- Fresh basil leaves

For the dressing...
- 1 tablespoon extra-virgin olive oil
- 1 1/2 teaspoons balsamic vinegar
- Honey, to taste
- Salt and pepper, to taste

Method:
1. Grab a medium bowl and add the arugula, tomato, avocado and mozzarella. Feel free to get creative and make it look pretty!
2. Top with basil leaves.
3. Grab a small bowl and add the olive oil, balsamic vinegar, sugar or honey and salt and pepper. Stir well to combine.
4. Pour the dressing over the salad, toss then serve and enjoy.

Quinoa and Kale Protein Power Salad

This protein-rich, gluten-free salad is one of my favorite lunchtime options in the world! Easy to take with you to the office and fancy enough to share at a bigger gathering, it combines fruits, nuts, beans, quinoa and green leafy veggies to create something astonishingly good.

Serves: 6
Time: 15 mins

- Calories: 453
- Net carbs: 68g
- Protein: 15g
- Fat: 14g

Ingredients:

- 2 cups cooked quinoa
- 2 cups chopped kale, ribs removed
- 1 x 15 oz. can garbanzo beans, drained
- 5-6 clementine oranges, peeled and sliced
- 1/3 cup chopped pistachios
- 1/3 cup pomegranate seeds
- 3 tablespoons extra virgin olive oil
- 1 tablespoon pomegranate molasses
- 1 tablespoon fresh orange juice
- 1 garlic clove, pressed or minced
- 2 teaspoons sumac, divided
- 1 teaspoon dried mint, crushed
- Salt and pepper, to taste
- 1/4 cup chopped fresh mint

Method:

1. Grab a large bowl and add the quinoa, kale, garbanzo beans, orange slices, pistachios and pomegranate seeds. Toss to combine.
2. Take a small bowl and add the olive oil, molasses, garlic, sumac, mint and seasonings. Stir well to combine.
3. Pour the dressing over the salad then toss again.
4. Serve with fresh mint and enjoy!

Greek Pasta Salad with Cucumbers & Artichoke Hearts

As a child, I was lucky enough to spend a lot of time in the Greek Islands. So whenever I sink my teeth into this amazing pasta salad I'm transported right back there and I can practically feel the sun on my back! I'm sure you'll love it too! Tangy cheese, salty olives and plenty of crunch. Mmmm....

Serves: 4-6
Time: 15 mins
- Calories: 557
- Net carbs: 82g
- Protein: 16g
- Fat: 18g

Ingredients:
- 1 lb. wholemeal pasta, cooked, drained and cooled
- 2 x 15 oz. cans quartered artichoke hearts in brine, drained
- 1 x 12 oz. jar roasted red bell peppers, slivered or chopped
- 1 x 8 oz. jar kalamata olives, halved
- 1 hot house cucumber, cut into 3/8" slices
- ¼ red onion, thinly sliced
- 1 cup crumbled feta cheese
- 1/3 cup fresh slivered or chopped basil leaves

For the dressing...
- ½ cup olive oil
- 1/4 cup white balsamic vinegar
- 4 cloves garlic, minced or pressed
- 2 tablespoons dry oregano
- Salt and pepper, to taste

Method:
1. Grab a large bowl and add the cooked pasta, artichoke, peppers, olives, cucumber, onion and half of the feta cheese. Toss to combine.
2. Find a smaller bowl and add the olive oil, vinegar, garlic, oregano and seasoning. Stir well to combine.
3. Pour over the salad and toss well to combine.
4. Top with the rest of the feta and extra basil leaves, season well then serve and enjoy!

Arugula Salad with Pesto Shrimp, Parmesan and Beans

Shrimp combines surprisingly well with basil pesto, white beans and parmesan. I'd go as far as to say that it's incredible. You will need to marinade the shrimp for best results, but if you're hungry and don't have much time, feel free to skip this step.

Serves: 2-4

Time: 15 mins (plus 30 mins to marinade + 30 minutes to rest, opt.)

- Calories: 574
- Net carbs: 79g
- Protein: 18g
- Fat: 23g

Ingredients:
- 8 oz. raw jumbo shrimp, peeled and deveined
- 4 tablespoons olive oil, divided
- 2 cloves garlic, pressed or minded
- Salt and pepper, to taste
- Pinch of red pepper flakes
- 2 cups cherry tomatoes
- 1/4 cup pesto
- 8 cups baby arugula
- 1/2 lemon
- 1/8 cup freshly shaved parmesan cheese
- 1/2 cup canned cannellini beans, rinsed and drained

Method:
1. Find a medium bowl and add the shrimp, olive oil, garlic, salt, pepper and garlic flakes.
2. Stir well then pop to one side for 30 minutes.
3. Place a skillet over a medium heat, add a tablespoon of the oil and heat.
4. Cook the shrimp, making sure they don't overlap. Flip after a minute or two.
5. Reduce the heat and add the remaining oil, garlic and tomatoes. Stir well to combine.
6. Remove the pan from the heat and place the shrimp into a medium bowl.
7. Add the pesto, stir well then pop to one side.
8. Find a large bowl, add the arugula and drizzle with the lemon juice. Stir well to combine.
9. Add the parmesan, beans and everything from the skillet.
10. Toss well to combine, season and leave to rest for 30 minutes before you serve and enjoy!

Autumn Couscous

Enjoy this colorful couscous as a side dish, a healthy snack or even a whole meal on its own. Packed with antioxidants, protein, healthy fats and flavor, it will keep your tummy satisfied whilst also filling any cravings for comfort foods.

Serves: 6
Time: 15 mins (plus 30 mins resting time, opt.)
- Calories: 387
- Net carbs: 67g
- Protein: 5g
- Fat: 13g

Ingredients:
- 8 oz. couscous, cooked
- 1 tablespoon olive oil
- 1 shallot, diced
- 1 fennel bulb, diced
- 2 ½ cups butternut squash, peeled, seeded and diced
- 3 tablespoons fresh sage, chopped
- ¾ cup dried cranberries
- ½ cup dried currants
- 1 ½ cups apple juice
- ¼ cup of the cooking juice (reserved from cooking the squash)
- ¼ cup olive oil
- 3 tablespoons red wine vinegar
- Salt and pepper, to taste
- 1 tablespoon parsley, chopped

Method:
1. Grab a large bowl and add the cooked couscous.
2. Place a pan over a medium heat and add the oil.
3. Add the shallot and fennel and cook for five minutes until soft.
4. Add the squash, sage, cranberries, currants and apple juice.
5. Cook for 15 minutes until the butternut squash softens, stirring often.
6. Season well then remove from the heat.
7. Drain about ¼ cup of the liquid to a measuring cup then transfer the veggies to the bowl with the couscous and stir through.
8. Take a small bowl, add the cooking liquid, oil, vinegar and seasoning. Stir well to combine.
9. Pour over the couscous and leave to rest for 30 minutes.
10. Toss well to combine then serve and enjoy!

Greek Salad with Avocado

Just one sentence is needed; best Greek salad in the world EVER!

Serves: 4
Time: 15 mins
- Calories: 833
- Net carbs: 39g
- Protein: 10g
- Fat: 73g

Ingredients:
- 2 English cucumbers, peeled in stripes and cut into ½" slices
- 1 1/2 lb. cherry tomatoes, stemmed and quartered
- 1/2 red onion, thinly sliced
- 1 1/2 cups Kalamata olives, pitted and halved
- 1/4 cup Italian flat leaf parsley, chopped
- 2 avocados, pitted and cut into chunks
- 1 cup feta cheese, broken into large chunks
- 1/2 cup extra virgin olive oil
- 1/2 cup red wine vinegar
- 2 cloves garlic, peeled and minced
- 1 tablespoon oregano
- 2 teaspoons sugar
- Salt and pepper, to taste

Method:
1. Grab a large bowl and add the tomatoes, cucumbers, onion, olives and parsley. Stir well to combine.
2. Take a small bowl, add the oil, vinegar, garlic, oregano, sugar and salt and pepper. Stir well to combine.
3. Place the avocado onto a small plate and pour a tablespoon of the dressing over the top.
4. Pour the remaining dressing mixture over the salad and toss to coat.
5. Place the avocado and feta over the top.
6. Serve and enjoy!

Garlicky Swiss Chard and Garbanzo Beans

This iron-rich warm salad is fabulous for those winter months when you want to maximize your veggie input but you need to stay warm. Soft, tender garbanzo beans, chard, fresh and salty feta and all the garlicky taste you could ever desire.

Serves: 2
Time: 20 mins
- Calories: 465
- Net carbs: 52g
- Protein: 25g
- Fat: 15g

Ingredients:
- 2 tablespoons olive oil, divided
- 2 bunches Swiss chard, chopped
- 2 cups chicken/vegetable broth or water
- 2 medium shallots, finely chopped
- 6 medium garlic cloves, minced
- 1 x 15 ½ oz. can garbanzo beans chickpeas, rinsed and drained
- 2 tablespoons freshly squeezed lemon juice
- Salt and pepper, to taste
- 1/2 cup crumbled feta cheese, optional

Method:
1. Grab a large skillet and add a tablespoon of the olive oil. Pop over a medium heat.
2. Add half the chard and cook for a minute or two until wilted. Add the remaining chard and repeat the process.
3. Add the chicken broth, cover and leave to cook for 10 minutes or so until tender.
4. Drain and pop the chard to one side.
5. Clean the skillet then add the remaining oil. Place back over the medium heat.
6. Add the shallots and garlic and cook for 5 minutes until soft.
7. Add the chard and chickpeas and cook again for another five minutes until heated through.
8. Transfer to a serving dish, squeeze the lemon juice over the top, sprinkle with cheese and season to taste.
9. Serve and enjoy!

Citrus Shrimp and Avocado Salad

The ingredients for this recipe might look like your grocery list but it's not as bad as it seems! Whip up the sauce, add the shrimp then create your salad. That's all it takes before you can fill up your belly with this light and nourishing salad. Delicious!

Serves: 4-6
Time: 25 mins
- Calories: 432
- Net carbs: 15g
- Protein: 37g
- Fat: 27g

Ingredients:

For the pan-search citrus shrimp...
- 1 teaspoon olive oil
- 1/3 cup fresh orange juice
- 3 tablespoons fresh lemon juice
- 1-2 garlic cloves, minced or pressed
- 1/8 red onion, finely chopped
- Fresh parsley, to taste
- Pinch of red pepper flakes
- Freshly ground black pepper and kosher salt
- 1 lb. medium shrimp, peeled and deveined
- Orange or lemon wedges, to taste

For the salad...
- 8 cups greens such as arugula spinach, or spring mix
- Extra virgin olive oil
- Juice of 1/2 lemon or 1/2 orange
- 1 avocado, sliced or diced
- 1 shallot, minced
- 4 oz. toasted sliced almonds
- Salt and pepper, to taste

Method:
1. Grab a medium bowl and add the olive oil, orange juice, lemon juice, garlic, onion, parsley and red pepper flakes. Stir well to combine.
2. Place into a skillet over a medium heat and bring to a simmer.
3. Cook for 5-10 minutes until reduces down to half.
4. Add the shrimp, season with salt and pepper and cook for a further 5 minutes.
5. Remove from the heat and leave to cool slightly.
6. Take a large bowl and add the salad greens.
7. Drizzle with oil and any remaining sauce from the shrimp.
8. Add the shrimp and toss well to combine.
9. Top with the avocado, shallots and sliced almonds, season well then serve and enjoy.

Mediterranean-Style Mustard Potato Salad

Just a warning- make this amazing potato salad and you will have crowds of people begging you for the recipe! Just get those potatoes cooked, throw your dressing ingredients together and you're practically done.

Serves: 6
Time: 21 mins
- Calories: 249
- Net carbs: 36g
- Protein: 9g
- Fat: 16g

Ingredients:
- 1 1/2 lb. baby potatoes, unpeeled and sliced thinly
- Water as needed
- 2 teaspoons salt
- 1/4 cup chopped red onions
- 1/4 cup fresh chopped parsley
- 1/4 cup chopped dill
- 2 tablespoons capers

For the dressing...
- 1/3 cup extra virgin olive oil
- 2 tablespoons white wine vinegar
- 2 teaspoons Dijon mustard
- 1/2 teaspoon ground sumac
- 1/2 teaspoon black pepper
- 1/4 teaspoon ground coriander

Method:
1. Grab a pan and add plenty of water. Add the potatoes and bring to a boil. Cook for 5-10 minutes until soft.
2. Drain and season well.
3. Season well then set to one side.
4. Find a medium bowl and add the dressing ingredients. Stir well to combine.
5. Add the potatoes and toss to coat.
6. Add the onions, fresh herbs and capers then toss again.
7. Place into a serving bowl and leave to rest for five minutes.
8. Serve and enjoy.

Herby Tuna Salad with Lime Dressing

Hands up if you're in the mood for a bowl of fresh flavors and epic crunch! I know I am. Providing everything your body needs to fuel your body and mind, you'll want to make this one regularly. Just sayin'.

Serves: 6
Time: 15 mins
- Calories: 175
- Net carbs: 14g
- Protein: 20g
- Fat: 7g

Ingredients:

For the lime dressing...
- 2 1/2 teaspoons Dijon mustard
- Zest of 1 lime
- Juice of 1 1/2 limes
- 1/3 cup extra virgin olive oil
- 1/2 teaspoon sumac
- Pinch of salt and pepper
- 1/2 teaspoon crushed red pepper flakes, optional

For the salad...
- 3 x 5 oz. cans tuna in olive oil
- 2 1/2 celery stalks, chopped
- 1/2 English cucumber, chopped
- 4-5 whole small radishes, stems removed, chopped
- 3 green onions, both white and green parts, chopped
- 1/2 medium-sized red onion, finely chopped
- 1/2 cup pitted Kalamata olives, halved
- 1 cup chopped fresh parsley
- 1/2 cup chopped fresh mint

To serve...
- 6 slices heirloom tomatoes
- Pitta chips or pitta pockets

Method:
1. First take a small bowl and add the vinaigrette ingredients. Stir well to combine then set to one side.
2. Grab a medium bowl and add the tuna, veggies, olives, parsley, and mint. Stir well to combine.
3. Add the vinaigrette and toss to combine.
4. Pop into the fridge for half an hour to rest then serve and enjoy

Soups

White Bean Soup

This is a simple and utterly delicious soup which my Italian grandmother used to make for me whenever I was sick. I don't know whether it was the garlic, the veggies or simply the comfort factor. But I promise you I felt amazing after eating a bowl or two of the stuff.

Serves: 6
Time: 35 mins
- Calories: 249
- Net carbs: 46g
- Protein: 15g
- Fat: 3g

Ingredients:
- 1 tablespoon olive oil
- 1 large onion, chopped
- 2 garlic cloves, minced
- 1 large carrot, chopped
- 1 celery rib, chopped
- 6 cups vegetable broth
- 1 teaspoon dried thyme
- ½ teaspoon oregano
- Salt and pepper, to taste
- 3 x 15 oz. cans white beans, drained and rinsed
- 2 cups baby spinach

To serve...
- Fresh parsley
- Grated parmesan cheese

Method:
1. Place a large saucepan over a medium heat and add the olive oil.
2. Throw in the onions and garlic and cook for a few minutes until soft.
3. Add the carrots, celery, thyme, oregano, salt and pepper and cook for a further five minutes.
4. Stir through the vegetable broth and beans and bring to a boil.
5. Reduce the heat and simmer for 15 minutes.
6. Turn off the heat and stir through the spinach.
7. Divide between serving bowls, sprinkle with parmesan and parsley.
8. Serve and enjoy!

Roasted Red Pepper and Tomato Soup

This gorgeous and satisfying gourmet soup does take slightly longer than most to make, but I promise that it's absolutely worth the effort. Sweet roasted red pepper, Italian herbs and punchy flavor make it far too moreish and perfect for sharing.

Makes: 4 cups
Time: 1 hour

- Calories: 99
- Net carbs: 11g
- Protein: 2g
- Fat: 5g

Ingredients:

- 2 red bell peppers, seeded and halved
- 3 tomatoes, cored and halved
- 1/2 medium onion, quartered
- 2 cloves garlic, peeled and halved
- 1-2 tablespoon olive oil
- Salt and pepper, to taste
- 2 cups vegetable broth
- 2 tablespoons tomato paste
- 1/4 cup fresh parsley, chopped
- 1/4 teaspoon Italian seasoning blend
- 1/4 teaspoon ground paprika
- 1/8 teaspoon ground cayenne pepper, or more to taste

Method:

1. Preheat your oven to 375°F and grease a baking tray.
2. Place the red pepper, tomato, onion and garlic onto the baking tray and drizzle with extra olive oil.
3. Season well then transfer to the oven and cook for 45 minutes until soft.
4. Remove from the oven and pop to one side.
5. Next take a medium pan and add the vegetable stock plus the roasted veggies, tomato paste, parsley, paprika and cayenne. Stir well.
6. Simmer for 10 minutes to allow the flavors to combine.
7. Using an immersion blender, whizz the soup down to your desired consistency.
8. Serve and enjoy!

Moroccan Lentil Soup

Lentils make a filling and nourishing base for any soup which provide useful levels of minerals, carbs and flavor. Teamed with garbanzo beans and veggies, and shaken up with spicy Moroccan spices, it's perfect for any hungry tummy!

Serves: 6-8
Time: 1 hour 5 mins
- Calories: 568
- Net carbs: 26g
- Protein: 14g
- Fat: 7.3g

Ingredients:
- 2 tablespoons extra virgin olive oil
- 1 large yellow onion, finely chopped
- 2 stalks celery, finely chopped
- 1 carrot, peeled and finely chopped
- 1/3 cup chopped parsley
- 1/2 cup chopped cilantro
- 5 large garlic cloves, chopped
- 2 tablespoons minced ginger
- 1 teaspoon ground turmeric
- 1 teaspoon ground cinnamon
- 2 teaspoons sweet paprika
- 1/2 teaspoon Aleppo pepper (opt.)
- 1 1/4 cups dry red lentils, rinsed and picked over
- 1 x 15 oz. can chickpeas, drained
- 1 x 28 oz. can chopped tomatoes
- 7–8 cups chicken broth or vegetable broth
- Coarse salt

To serve...
- Dates,
- Lemon wedges

Method:
1. Take a large pan, add the olive oil and place over a medium heat.
2. Add the onion, celery, carrots, garlic and ginger and cook for 5 minutes until soft.
3. Throw in the spices and stir again. Cook for a further 2 minutes.
4. Next add the tomatoes and the broth and bring to a simmer.
5. Add the lentils, chickpeas, cilantro and parsley and simmer for 35 minutes until the lentils break down.
6. Season well then serve and enjoy.

Greek Lemon Chicken Soup

Light and refreshing yet filling and nourishing, this chicken soup is amazing. If you're not a fan of couscous you can replace with rice and adjust the cooking time and method accordingly. Feel free to throw in whatever veggies you like if you want to get creative. Spinach and kale work brilliantly.

Serves: 8
Time: 30 mins
- Calories: 214
- Net carbs: 22g
- Protein: 11g
- Fat: 8g

Ingredients:
- 10 cups chicken broth
- 3 tablespoons olive oil
- 8 cloves garlic, minced
- 1 sweet onion, finely chopped
- 1 large lemon, zested
- 2 boneless skinless chicken breasts
- 1 cup Israeli couscous
- 1/2 teaspoon crushed red pepper
- 2 oz. crumbled feta
- 1/3 cup chopped chive
- Salt and pepper, to taste

Method:
1. Take a large pan, add the olive oil and place over a medium heat.
2. Add the onion and garlic and cook for 5 minutes until soft.
3. Add the broth, chicken breasts, lemon zest and crushed pepper.
4. Cover and bring to a boil, then reduce the heat and simmer for five minutes.
5. Stir through the couscous, season well and cook for a further five minutes.
6. Remove from the heat and carefully remove the chicken from the pot.
7. Using two forks shred the chicken and place back into the pot.
8. Stir through the feta and olives, season well, then serve and enjoy.

Minestrone Soup

Mmmmm.... this amazing Minestrone soup leaves me speechless!! Pile in the white beans, red beans, wholemeal pasta, tomatoes and a gorgeous collection of herbs and you have something that will keep you fueled for practically anything!!

Serves: 8
Time: 1 hour 20 mins
- Calories: 309
- Net carbs: 44g
- Protein: 16g
- Fat: 9g

Ingredients:
- 1 small white onion, minced
- 4 cloves garlic, minced
- ½ cup sliced carrots
- 1 medium zucchini, sliced, then cut slices in half
- 1 medium yellow squash, sliced, then cut slices in half
- 2 tablespoons minced fresh parsley
- ¼ cup celery, sliced
- 3 tablespoons extra olive oil
- 2 x 15 oz. cannellini beans, rinsed and drained
- 2 x 15 oz. red kidney beans, rinsed and drained
- 1 x 14.5 oz. fire-roasted diced tomatoes, drained
- 4 cups vegetable stock
- 2 cups water
- 1½ teaspoon oregano
- ½ teaspoon basil
- ¼ teaspoon thyme
- 1 teaspoon salt
- ½ teaspoon pepper
- ¾ cup small wholemeal pasta shells
- 4 cups fresh baby spinach
- ¼ cup Parmesan or Romano cheese

Method:
1. Place a large pan over a medium heat and add the oil.
2. Throw in the onions, garlic, carrots, zucchini, squash, parsley and celery. Cook for five minutes until soft.
3. Throw in the stock, water, cannellini beans, kidney beans, tomatoes, herbs, salt and pepper.
4. Bring to a boil then reduce the heat and simmer for 20-30 minutes until the vegetables are soft.
5. Remove from the heat and stir through the cheese.
6. Serve and enjoy.

Simple Zucchini & Garlic Soup

Who says you need to use dairy to enjoy an amazingly creamy zucchini soup? With just a handful of ingredients and a ton of love, you can create this tasty soup and have it on the table fast.

Serves: 8
Time: 30 mins
- Calories: 62
- Net carbs: 5g
- Protein: 3g
- Fat: 4g

Ingredients:
- 2 ½ lb. zucchini
- 1 medium onion, diced
- 2 tablespoons olive oil
- 4 garlic cloves, chopped
- 4 cups chicken stock or broth
- Sea salt and pepper, to taste
- ⅓ cup fresh basil leaves

Method:
1. Grab a medium pan, add the oil and place over a medium heat.
2. Add the onion, zucchini and garlic and cook for five minutes.
3. Add the stock and simmer for another 15 minutes.
4. Remove from the heat, season well and stir through the basil leaves.
5. Using an immersion blender, puree the soup to taste.
6. Serve and enjoy.

Chicken Leek Soup with White Wine

1. Straight from the island of Crete, this is a delicious soup that sits light in your stomach so you can enjoy yourself in the sun without feeling weighed down. Perfect teamed with a glass of wine, and even tastier when enjoyed al fresco, it's flavor-rich and full of healthy protein. If you'd prefer to avoid the wine, just switch for broth.

Serves: 5
Time: 50 mins

- Calories: 576
- Net carbs: 9g
- Protein: 57g
- Fat: 31g

Ingredients:

- 1/2 cup extra virgin olive oil
- 2 lb. chicken breast, cut into bite-sized pieces
- 1 large leek, cut into thin rounds
- 4 green onions, chopped
- 4 celery sticks, chopped
- 1 small cabbage, cut into thick slices
- 1 cup white wine
- Salt and pepper, to taste
- 1/2 teaspoon paprika
- Pinch of nutmeg
- 3 cups water

Method:

1. Grab a large pan, pop over a medium heat and add the olive oil.
2. Throw in the chicken and stir until cooked outside.
3. Add the leeks, green onions and celery and cook for a further minute.
4. Add the cabbage and cook for another minute or so.
5. Pour in the wine and water and add the salt, pepper, paprika, nutmeg and water. Stir well to combine.
6. Cover with the lid and simmer for 45 minutes until perfectly cooked.
7. Serve and enjoy.

Italian Meatball Soup

Although you absolutely could use pre-made meatballs, you'd be reducing the benefits of the diet and also missing out on a ton of fun. Besides, they're super easy to make, so no excuses. Enjoy!

Serves: 3
Time: 40 mins
- Calories: 582
- Net carbs: 25g
- Protein: 42g
- Fat: 36g

Ingredients:

For the meatballs...
- 1 lb. ground beef
- 1/4 - 1/2 cup freshly grated parmesan cheese, optional
- 1 free-range egg
- 1 cup breadcrumbs (opt.)
- 2 tablespoons fresh parsley, minced
- 1 teaspoon dried oregano
- 1/2 teaspoon sea salt

For the soup...
- ½ teaspoon black pepper
- 3 tablespoons olive oil
- 2 quarts chicken broth or beef broth
- 3 tablespoons tomato paste
- 1 onion, diced
- 2 bay leaves
- 4-5 sprigs fresh thyme
- ½ teaspoon whole black peppercorns
- Fresh parmesan cheese, grated
- 1-2 tablespoons fresh basil leaves, torn
- 1-2 tablespoons fresh parsley, chopped
- Salt and pepper, to taste

Method:
1. Grab a medium bowl and add the meatball ingredients. Stir well then shape into small balls with your hands.
2. Place a medium pan over a medium heat and add the oil.
3. Cook the meatballs until brown then pop to one side.
4. Use a wooden spoon to scrape off any stuck bits then add the soup ingredients, stirring well to combine.
5. Cover with the lid then bring to the boil.
6. Reduce the heat to a simmer and cook for 5-10 minutes until everything is sort.

7. Add the meatballs to the pan, simmer for a couple more minutes then remove from the heat.
8. Serve and enjoy.

Greek Easter Lamb Soup

This is another very traditional Greek soup which comes straight from my grandmother. Usually eaten on Easter Sunday, it boasts a unique and flavorsome combination of dill, green onions, lettuce, eggs and lamb plus just the right amount of olive oil. But don't worry- it doesn't need to be Easter for you to enjoy it.

Serves: 5
Time: 1 hour 40 mins
- Calories: 710
- Net carbs: 3g
- Protein: 42g
- Fat: 58g

Ingredients:
- 1/2 cup extra virgin olive oil
- 2 lb. lamb, cut into bite-sized pieces
- 10 green onions, chopped
- 5 cups water
- 2 bunches dill, chopped
- 1 head romaine lettuce, chopped very thin
- Salt and pepper, to taste
- Juice of 3 lemons
- 3 free-range eggs

Method:
1. Place a large pan over a medium heat and add the oil.
2. Add the lamb and any bones, and sauté for 10 minutes, stirring often.
3. Throw in the onions and sauté for another 5 minutes.
4. Add the water, stir well then cover with the lid.
5. Bring to a boil then simmer for 30 minutes.
6. Add the lettuce, dill, salt and pepper then simmer for a further hour. Remove from the heat.
7. Meanwhile, find a small bowl and whisk together the eggs and lemon juice.
8. Carefully ladle a small amount of the soup broth into the egg mixture, stirring constantly. Add a second ladle of the broth and do the same.
9. Pour the egg mixture into the soup and stir through carefully.
10. Serve and enjoy!

Tuscan White Bean Soup with Sausage and Kale

What do you get if you combine gorgeous Italian sausage, tender white beans, fresh mineral-rich chard and fragrant garlic? Gorgeous eaten in front of a fire on a cold winter's day, it's guaranteed to put a smile on your face.

Serves: 6
Time: 20 mins
- Calories: 867
- Net carbs: 87g
- Protein: 41g
- Fat: 23g

Ingredients:
- ¼ cup extra-virgin olive oil
- 1 lb. hot or sweet Italian sausage, cut into bite sized pieces
- 1 onion, chopped
- 1 carrot, chopped
- 1 stalk celery, chopped
- 2 cloves garlic, chopped
- ½ lb. kale, stems removed and chopped
- 4 cups chicken broth
- 1 x 8 oz. can cannelloni beans, rinsed and drained
- 1 teaspoon rosemary, dried
- 1 bay leaf
- ¼ teaspoon pepper
- Salt, to taste
- ½ cup shredded Parmesan

Method:
1. Place a large pan over a medium heat and add the olive oil.
2. Add the sausage and cook until browned on all sides.
3. Throw in the onion, carrot, celery and garlic and cook for a further 5 minutes until soft.
4. Add the kale and stir well until wilted.
5. Add the broth, beans, rosemary and bay leaf, stir well then cover with the lid
6. Bring to a boil then reduce the heat and simmer for 30 minutes.
7. Serve and enjoy.

Sandwiches & Wraps

Mediterranean Tuna Sandwiches

Light up your lunchtime with these healthy tuna sandwiches. Although the recipe contains mayo, feel free to substitute with a drop of olive oil, hummus or tzatziki and take it to a whole new level of awesome.

Serves: 4
Time: 15 mins
- Calories: 293
- Net carbs: 31g
- Protein: 21g
- Fat: 10g

Ingredients:
- 4 teaspoons olive oil
- 4 teaspoons red wine vinegar
- 8 slices whole-grain bread
- 2 x 6 oz. cans low-sodium tuna in water, drained and flaked
- 1/3 cup sun-dried tomato halves in olive, drained and chopped
- 1/4 cup sliced ripe olives
- 1/4 cup finely chopped red onion
- 3 tablespoons mayonnaise
- 2 teaspoons capers
- 1/4 teaspoon freshly ground black pepper
- 4 romaine lettuce leaves

Method:
1. Take a small bowl and add the olive oil and vinegar. Stir well to combine.
2. Brush the oil mixture over one side of each bread slice.
3. Take another bowl and add the tuna, sundried tomatoes, olives, red onion, mayonnaise, capers and pepper. Stir well to combine.
4. Place a lettuce leaf onto each slice of bread, top with the tuna, spread well then top with the other slice of bread.
5. Slice then serve and enjoy.

Avocado Feta Wrap

When you need to prepare a quick lunch but you barely have a minute to space, grab some avocado, feta and something green and leafy and you'll create something awesome. Trust me.

Serves: 2
Time: 10 mins
- Calories: 548
- Net carbs: 37g
- Protein: 18g
- Fat: 38g

Ingredients:
- 2 x 10" wraps or tortillas (plain or flavored)
- ½ cup feta cheese
- 1 medium ripe avocado, cut into strips
- 1 tablespoon lemon juice
- 1 tablespoon olive oil
- 1 cup rocket salad leaves

Method:
1. Take a medium bowl and add the olive oil and lemon juice. Stir well to combine.
2. Add the rocket leaves and toss to coat in the dressing.
3. Place the wraps onto a flat surface and add the rocket, cheese and avocado strips, concentrating the filling in the center.
4. Roll up, slice then serve and enjoy.

Pesto Goat Cheese Eggplant Wrap

Talk about special! This eggplant wrap combines the best in Mediterranean flavors to create something that will wow your taste buds. If you're prefer, you can roast the eggplant at home to reduce the oil and up the flavor. The choice is yours.

Serves: 2
Time: 10 mins
- Calories: 810
- Net carbs: 93g
- Protein: 16g
- Fat: 27g

Ingredients:
- 2 x 10" wraps or tortillas
- 4-6 tablespoons pesto sauce
- ¼ cup roasted eggplant preserved in oil, drained and cut into strips
- ½ cup fresh goat cheese, chopped
- 1 cup rocket salad leaves

Method:
1. Place the wraps onto a flat surface and spread with the pesto sauce.
2. Place the eggplant onto the wraps, followed by the cheese and rocket.
3. Roll up, slice then serve and enjoy.

Mediterranean Hummus Wrap

Hummus is a brilliantly versatile dip or spread that you can use as a base for any sandwich or wrap. Throw in whatever salad veggies you can and get eating!

Serves: 2
Time: 10 mins
- Calories: 879
- Net carbs: 76g
- Protein: 46g
- Fat: 86g

Ingredients:
- 2 x 10" wraps or tortillas
- ½ cup hummus
- 2 large-sized lettuce leaves
- ¼ cup roasted red peppers, drained
- ¼ cup Greek olives, pitted
- ¼ cup sundried tomatoes, drained
- ½ cup shredded Emmental cheese

Method:
1. Place the wraps onto a flat surface and spread the hummus over each wrap.
2. Cover with the lettuce leaf, top with the peppers, olives, tomatoes and cheese.
3. Roll up, slice and then serve and enjoy.

Mediterranean Chicken Wraps with Hummus

More hummus, but this time combined with chicken, olives and whatever other ingredients you can squeeze in! Remember- this is your wrap so make it exactly as you want it to be.

Serves: 6
Time: 10 mins
- Calories: 356
- Net carbs: 38g
- Protein: 19g
- Fat: 11g

Ingredients:
- 2 chicken breasts, cooked and sliced
- 10 oz. cherry tomatoes, halved
- 1 small red onion, chopped
- 1 large cucumber, peeled and diced
- 3 tablespoons red wine vinegar
- 1 tablespoon olive oil
- 1/2 teaspoon salt
- 1/2 teaspoon fresh black pepper
- 2 cups shredded romaine lettuce
- 1/2 cup jarred pepperoncini, drained of excess liquid
- 1 can black olives, roughly chopped
- 1 jar artichoke hearts, drained and quartered
- 1/2 cup feta cheese, crumbled
- 1 cup hummus
- 6 fresh tortilla wraps

Method:
1. Grab a large bowl and add the tomatoes, onion, cucumber, vinegar, olive oil, salt and pepper. Stir to combine then pop to one side.
2. Place the wraps onto a flat surface and spread with the hummus.
3. Top with chicken, lettuce, tomato, pepperoncinis, olives, artichokes and feta.
4. Roll up, slice and then serve and enjoy.

Easy Chicken Sandwiches

Forget whatever you think a chicken sandwich needs to be like and create this one instead! It will light up your taste buds, fill up your tummy and make you say 'Wow'. The secret lies in the herbs so please don't skip.

Serves: 6
Time: 20 mins
- Calories: 227
- Net carbs: 22g
- Protein: 26g
- Fat: 4g

Ingredients:
- 1 1/4 lb. boneless skinless chicken breasts, cut into 1-inch strips
- 2 medium tomatoes, seeded and chopped
- 1/2 cup sliced quartered seeded cucumber
- 1/2 cup sliced sweet onion
- 2 tablespoons cider vinegar
- 1 tablespoon olive oil
- 1 teaspoon dried oregano
- 1/2 teaspoon dried mint
- 1/4 teaspoon salt

To taste...
- 6 whole wheat pita pocket halves, warmed
- 6 lettuce leaves

Method:
1. Take a large skillet, add the oil and place over a medium heat.
2. Add the chicken and cook for five minutes until cooked.
3. Remove from the pan and pop to one side.
4. Grab a large bowl, add the chicken, tomatoes, cucumber and onion and stir well.
5. Take a small bowl and add the vinegar, oil, oregano, mint and salt. Stir well to combine.
6. Pour the dressing over the chicken mixture and toss to coat.
7. Pop into the fridge for an hour to allow the flavors to combine.
8. Open up the pitta pockets, fill with the chicken mixture then serve and enjoy.

Falafel Pitta Sandwich

Falafel are the taste of the Middle East which provides plenty of plant-based, vegan-friendly protein and hits that comfort food factor. You can also bake the falafel if you'd prefer, but I highly recommend frying for best results.

Serves: 6
Time: 15 mins
- Calories: 227
- Net carbs: 41g
- Protein: 9g
- Fat: 3g

Ingredients:
For the falafel...
- 1 x 16 oz. can garbanzo beans
- 1 large onion, chopped
- 2 cloves garlic, chopped
- 3 tablespoons fresh parsley, chopped
- 1 teaspoon coriander
- 1 teaspoon cumin
- 2 tablespoons flour
- Salt and pepper, to taste
- Olive oil (for frying)

For the pittas...
- 6 pita bread loaves
- 2 tomatoes, diced
- 1 cucumber, diced
- 1 onion sliced, red or white
- 1/4 cup fresh parsley, finely chopped
- Tahini
- 1/4 cup sandwich pickles (opt.)

Method:
1. Grab a food processor and add the garbanzo beans, garlic, onion, coriander, cumin, flour and salt and pepper.
2. Hit that whizz button until the falafel mixture comes together.
3. Using your hands, form into balls.
4. Heat a small amount of oil in a skillet and fry the falafel until golden. Pop to one side.
5. Meanwhile warm the pittas in a microwave for a few moments then slice.
6. Fill the pockets with the falafel, tomatoes, cucumber, onion and parsley. Drizzle with tahini.
7. Serve and enjoy.

Mediterranean Veggie Sandwich with Smoked Tofu

Just because you're a vegetarian or vegan, that doesn't mean that you have to sacrifice the best flavors or textures of Mediterranean food. Whip out your grill or head outdoors for an authentic, totally amazing sandwich that tastes great.

Serves: 2
Time: 15 mins
- Calories: 246
- Net carbs: 33g
- Protein: 15g
- Fat: 4g

Ingredients:
- 2 rustic white artisan bread rolls
- 1/2 eggplant, sliced
- 1/2 zucchini, sliced
- 1 portobello mushroom, sliced
- 1/2 block smoked tofu, sliced
- Extra virgin olive oil
- Salt and pepper, to taste

Method:
1. Place the eggplant, zucchini, mushrooms and smoked tofu onto a flat surface and brush with the olive oil.
2. Season well then pop under a broiler until done.
3. Slice the bread rolls and brush with olive oil. Pop under the broiler and toast too.
4. Place the veggies and tofu onto the bread rolls, top with the other piece of the roll then serve and enjoy!

Hummus and Vegetable Sandwich

With just the right combination of veggies and a dollop of hummus, you can make the perfect sandwich that is a cut above the rest. If you can, we highly recommend the sourdough bread for the best flavor in the entire universe. Yum!

Serves: 1
Time: 10 mins
- Calories: 273
- Net carbs: 39g
- Protein: 6.9g
- Fat: 6g

Ingredients:
- 1 tablespoon hummus
- 1/2 medium zucchini, sliced thin lengthwise
- 1 small cucumber, sliced thin lengthwise
- 2 to 3 thin slices red onion
- Baby spinach
- 1 medium tomato, sliced thin
- 1 1/2 teaspoons feta or goat cheese crumbles
- 4 to 5 chopped Kalamata olives
- 2 slices whole grain sourdough bread

Method:
1. Place one slice of bread onto a flat surface and spread with the hummus.
2. Place the veggies on top of the hummus in layers, leaving the tomato to last.
3. Cover with cheese and olives and top with the other slice of bread.
4. Slice, serve and enjoy.

Mediterranean Black Olive Hummus Paninis

If you've never tried black olive hummus before, drop everything now and make this sandwich. It's salty, creamy and oh-so good, and when you team that with spinach, pepper and yet more olives...wow, simply wow....

Serves: 4
Time: 20 mins
- Calories: 592
- Net carbs: 73g
- Protein: 23g
- Fat: 28g

Ingredient:

For the black olive hummus...
- 1 x 14 oz. can garbanzo beans, drained and rinsed
- 2 tablespoons olive oil
- 2 tablespoons lemon juice
- 2 tablespoons tahini
- 1 tablespoon red wine vinegar
- 1/4 cup chopped fresh parsley
- 1 cup large black olives
- 1 tablespoon capers
- Black pepper, to taste

For the sandwich...
- 8 slices whole grain sandwich bread
- 1 cup fresh baby spinach
- 1/2 cup roasted red pepper, sliced
- 12 to 16 large black olives, sliced
- Extra virgin olive oil

Method:
1. Grab a food processor and add all the black olive hummus ingredients. Whizz until smooth.
2. Place half of the bread slices onto a flat surface and spread with some of the black olive hummus.
3. Cover with the spinach, red pepper slices and the olive slices.
4. Top with the other slice of bread.
5. Place a skillet over a medium heat and add some olive oil.
6. Place the sandwich into the skillet and toast on both sides until brown.
7. Slice, serve and enjoy.

Mediterranean Turkey Panini

This turkey panini sandwich is better than any other turkey sandwich you've tried in your entire life. The secret lies in the garlic aioli so be sure to slather your bread in as much of it as you like. The recipe I've included makes plenty so you can pop any leftovers in the fridge and use it to pimp your sandwiches for the rest of the week. You're welcome.

Serves: 1
Time: 15 mins

- Calories: 887
- Net carbs: 45g
- Protein: 37g
- Fat: 46g

Ingredients:

For the sandwich...

- 1 panini or other crusty bread
- 1 fresh tomato, sliced
- Fresh spinach leaves
- 1 oz. feta, crumbled
- 3 slices deli turkey
- Dash of salt and pepper

For the garlic aioli...

- 2 cloves garlic, minced
- 1/2 cup mayo
- 1/8 teaspoon salt
- 1/4 tablespoon lemon juice

Method:

1. Take a small bowl and add the minced garlic and salt. Stir well together then add the mayo and lemon juice.
2. Stir again then pop into the fridge to rest.
3. Place a grill pan over a medium heat and add oil if required.
4. Meanwhile, place the panini on a flat surface and layer with turkey, spinach, tomato, feta and salt and pepper.
5. Close and transfer to the grill to brown.
6. Slice then serve and enjoy.

Italian Panini Grill Sandwich

This is probably the most 'traditional' of all panini sandwiches in this book, and boy is it awesome! Flavor-rich red peppers, sweet roasted garlic and gorgeously melty mozzarella cheese come together to make this a sandwich fit for a king (or queen). Enjoy.

Serves: 2
Time: 10 mins

- Calories: 327
- Net carbs: 29g
- Protein: 8g
- Fat: 3g

Ingredients:

- 8 slices mozzarella cheese
- 1/4 cup roasted red peppers
- 4 canned artichoke slices
- 6 cloves roasted garlic
- 2 teaspoons olive oil
- 2 paninis (or your favorite bread)
- 1 teaspoon butter

Method:

1. Preheat your panini grill or broiler to 350°F.
2. Place the paninis onto a flat surface and spread with the butter.
3. Place into the grill with the butter side down until browned.
4. Remove from the grill and spread with the roasted garlic.
5. Top with two slices of cheese, roasted pepper and artichoke slices.
6. Add two more slices of cheese, cover with the other half of the panini and place back into the broiler.
7. Grill until the cheese has melted.
8. Slice then serve and enjoy.

Avocado Caprese Wrap

The classic Caprese salad can also be transformed into a satisfying and delicious wrap which will fill your stomach and keep you fueled through the rest of the afternoon. Keep it simple and enjoy how good it tastes.

Serves: 1-2
Time: 10 mins
- Calories: 645
- Net carbs: 72g
- Protein: 16g
- Fat: 41g

Ingredients:
- 2 whole wheat tortillas
- 1/2 cup fresh arugula leaves
- 1 ball fresh mozzarella cheese, sliced
- 1 tomato, sliced
- 1 avocado, pitted and sliced
- Basil leaves
- Extra virgin olive oil
- Balsamic vinegar
- Salt and pepper, to taste

Method:
1. Place the tortillas onto a flat surface.
2. Add the mozzarella, avocado, tomato slices and basil.
3. Drizzle with oil and vinegar then season well.
4. Roll up, slice then serve and enjoy.

Chicken & Turkey

Grilled Balsamic Chicken with Olive Tapenade

You won't believe the flavors that burst onto your taste buds when you try this grilled chicken recipe. Although it might seem like there's a huge list of ingredients, you needn't worry. Just throw the tapenade into your food processor and most of the hard work is done already.

Makes: 3 cups
Time: 10 mins
- Calories: 628
- Net carbs: 8g
- Protein: 70g
- Fat: 34g

Ingredients:
For the chicken...
- 2 chicken breasts
- 1/4 cup olive oil
- 1/4 cup balsamic vinegar
- 1/8 cup wholegrain garlic mustard
- 1 1/2 tablespoons balsamic vinegar
- 3 cloves garlic, pressed or minced
- Juice of 1/2 lemon
- 1 tablespoon fresh rosemary or thyme, chopped
- Salt and pepper to taste

For the olive tapenade...
- 3 cloves garlic, pressed or minced
- 1/4 cup olive oil
- 1/2 cup sun dried tomatoes, drained and coarsely chopped
- 1 x 4 oz. jar green olives, drained and pitted
- 1 x 6 oz. jar mixed Greek olives, drained and pitted
- Juice of 1 lemon
- 2 teaspoons balsamic vinegar
- 1/2 teaspoon freshly ground black pepper
- 1/3 cup fresh chopped parsley

Method:
1. Grab a food processor and add the garlic and olive oil. Whizz until blended.
2. Add the sundried tomatoes and whizz until chopped.
3. Add both types of olives and whizz until the olives are chopped (but not pureed!)
4. Throw in the lemon juice, vinegar, pepper, parsley and stir well.
5. Pop into the fridge until needed.
6. Grab a large bowl and add the olive oil, balsamic vinegar, mustard, garlic, lemon juice, herbs, and salt and pepper. Stir well to combine.

7. Pour half the marinade into a jug and add the chicken to the remaining marinade in the bowl. Leave for at least 30 minutes to marinade.
8. Preheat the broiler or grill to 400°F.
9. Remove the chicken from the marinade, brush with oil and place onto the grill until cooked, turning often. Baste with the remaining marinade as needed.
10. When cooked, place onto a serving dish and leave to rest for five minutes.
11. Serve with the tapenade plus feta cheese, herbs and extra oil.
12. Enjoy!

Greek Chicken Marinade

Garlicky, lemony and packed with gorgeously fragrant oregano, you can cook this chicken recipe whichever way you want and know that you'll have a happy crowd afterwards. It's also super simple to make and perfect for eating with a loved one or a group of friends.

Serves: 4
Time: 45 mins
- Calories: 268
- Net carbs: 6g
- Protein: 26g
- Fat: 17g

Ingredients:
- 1 lb. boneless skinless chicken breasts
- ⅓ cup plain Greek yogurt
- ¼ cup olive oil
- Juice of 4 lemons
- Zest of one lemon
- 4-5 cloves garlic, pressed or minced
- 2 tablespoons dried oregano
- Salt and pepper, to taste

Method:
1. Grab a medium bowl and add all the ingredients except for the chicken.
2. Stir well to combine then remove half of the mixture and pop to one side.
3. Add the chicken, stir to combine then pop into the fridge to marinade.
4. Preheat your broiler or grill to 400°F.
5. Remove the chicken from the marinade and cook for 20-30 minutes until cooked through.
6. Baste as required with the retained marinade.
7. Serve and enjoy.

Chicken Quinoa Bowl with Broccoli & Tomato

This protein rich meal is perfect for dinner and brilliant for eating at lunchtime when you really want to refuel. Although we'd suggested broccoli as the veggies in this dish, feel free to sub for whatever takes your fancy. Peppers, roasted garlic and olives are also awesome.

Serves: 2
Time: 30 mins
- Calories: 861
- Net carbs: 76g
- Protein: 29g
- Fat: 33g

Ingredients:

For the chicken...
- 1 x 6 oz. skinless, boneless chicken breast
- 1/4 cup olive oil plus 2 tablespoons
- 1 lemon, juiced and zested
- 2 cloves garlic, pressed or minced
- 2 teaspoons dried oregano
- Salt and pepper, to taste
- 3/4 cup cooked broccoli
- ¼ cup feta cheese, crumbled
- 1/2 cup pre-roasted tomatoes

For the quinoa...
- 1 cup dried quinoa
- Salt, to taste
- Feta cheese, crumbled

Method:
1. Take a medium bowl and add the ¼ cup olive oil, lemon juice and zest, garlic, oregano, salt and pepper. Stir well to combine.
2. Add the chicken, stir to cover then pop into the fridge to marinade for at least 30 minutes, preferably overnight.
3. When ready to cook, place the remaining oil into a skillet and pop over a medium heat.
4. Remove the chicken from the marinade and cook for 10-15 minutes, turning often as required.
5. Reduce the heat and add the broccoli and tomatoes and warm gently.
6. Cook the quinoa according to the instructions on the package.
7. Serve the quinoa and the chicken together then enjoy!

Greek Chicken Kebab

There's something about kebabs that always makes me think of the summer. I just want to head outdoors with my friends and loved ones, soak up the sun and enjoy everything that the better weather has to offer. And so will you.

Serves: 6
Time: 55 mins
- Calories: 194
- Net carbs: 8g
- Protein: 11g
- Fat: 18g

Ingredients:
- 1 lb. boneless skinless chicken breasts
- 1/3 cup plain Greek yogurt
- 1/4 cup olive oil
- Juice of 4 lemons
- Zest of a lemon
- 4-5 cloves garlic, pressed or minced
- 2 tablespoons dried oregano
- Salt and pepper, to taste
- 1 red onion, quartered
- 1 small zucchini, sliced
- 1 red bell pepper, cut into 1" pieces

Method:
1. Grab a large bowl and add the yoghurt, olive oil and zest and juice of one lemon. Stir well to combine.
2. Add the garlic, oregano, and seasoning and stir to combine.
3. Remove half the marinade and pop to one side then place the chicken into the remaining marinade in the bowl.
4. Stir well to coat then pop into the fridge to marinate for at least 30 minutes.
5. Preheat the broiler.
6. Remove the chicken from the fridge then thread onto skewers, alternating with the red onion, zucchini and red bell pepper.
7. Baste the kebabs with the marinade and broil for 10-15 minutes until cooked.
8. Serve and enjoy.

Quick Caprese Chicken

To make this epic chicken recipe, you simply need a pan, some great-quality ingredients and plenty of love. Simple, quick and tasty, you'll love it.

Serves: 2
Time: 30 mins
- Calories: 622
- Net carbs: 3g
- Protein: 80g
- Fat: 33g

Ingredients:
- 2 skinless boneless chicken breasts
- Salt and pepper, to taste
- 1 tablespoon extra-virgin olive oil
- 1 tablespoon butter
- 1 jar pesto
- 6 oz. grated mozzarella cheese
- 8 cocktail or small tomatoes, sliced

To serve...
- Balsamic vinegar
- Fresh basil, slivered

Method:
1. Preheat your oven to 400°F.
2. Slice the chicken breasts in half lengthwise then season well.
3. Grab a skillet and place over a medium heat. Add the olive oil and butter.
4. Add the chicken and cook for a few minutes on both sides.
5. Dollop around a tablespoon or so of pesto onto each piece of chicken, top with the mozzarella and tomato then place into the oven.
6. Cook for 10-12 minutes then remove from the oven.
7. Serve and enjoy with fresh basil and balsamic vinegar.

Grilled Greek Lemon Chicken Skewers

More kebabs for that summer experience, but this time infused with the uplifting and citrussy taste of lemon, oregano and plenty of garlic. For best results, we highly recommend that you marinate these ones, but feel free to skip if you're short on time.

Serves: 2
Time: 30 mins (plus 30 mins to marinade, opt.)
- Calories: 480
- Net carbs: 12g
- Protein: 42g
- Fat: 32g

Ingredients
- 2 boneless chicken breasts, cut into 1" chunks
- Juice of 2 lemons
- Zest of 1 lemon
- 4 cloves garlic, minced
- 1 tablespoon dried oregano
- 1/4 cup olive oil
- Salt and pepper, to taste
- 7-8 green onions, chopped

Method:
1. Preheat the broiler or grill to 400°F.
2. Grab a large bowl and add the lemon juice and zest, garlic, oregano, olive oil and seasoning. Stir well to combine.
3. Throw in the chicken and stir again to coat.
4. Cover and pop into the fridge for at least 30 minutes to marinade.
5. Remove the chicken from the fridge and thread onto skewers, alternating with the lemon slices, and green onions.
6. Pop under the grill and cook until the chicken is brown- about 10-15 minutes.
7. Serve and enjoy!

Greek Turkey Burgers with Tzatziki Sauce

Be ready to be wowed! These turkey burgers combine garlic, spinach, oregano, sundried tomatoes and feta cheese to create a dish that will leave you amazed and keep your tummy filled. You HAVE to try them. Seriously.

Serves: 4
Time: (30 mins, plus 30 mins resting time)
- Calories: 328
- Net carbs: 34g
- Protein: 37g
- Fat: 18g

Ingredients:
For the turkey burgers…
- 1 lb. ground turkey
- ½ cup fresh spinach leaves, chopped
- ⅓ cup sun-dried tomatoes, chopped
- 1/4 cup red onion, minced
- ¼ cup feta cheese, crumbled
- 2 cloves garlic, pressed or minced
- 1 free-range egg, whisked
- 1 tablespoon olive oil plus extra for frying
- 1 teaspoon dried oregano
- Salt and pepper, to taste

To serve…
- 4 soft whole-wheat hamburger buns
- Lettuce leaves
- Sliced red onion
- Tzatziki (recipe available in Dips & Spreads in this book)

Method:
1. Grab a large bowl and add the turkey, spinach, sundried tomatoes, red onion and feta. Stir well to combine.
2. Take a small bowl and add the garlic, egg, olive oil, oregano and seasoning then whisk together.
3. Pour over the meat mixture and combine well.
4. Using your hands, form into four burgers then pop into the fridge for 30 minutes to rest.
5. Pop a skillet over a medium heat and add a drop of oil.
6. Place the turkey burgers into the pan and cook until browned, flipping halfway through serving.
7. Serve with the lettuce leaves, red onion, bread rolls and tzatziki.
8. Enjoy!

One-Skillet Tomato and Olive Chicken

If you want to create a dish to impress, but you don't have hours to spend in the kitchen, give this tomato-olive chicken a try. The perfect one-pan meal, it's packed with protein, full of antioxidants and will help keep your waistline in check without you ever feeling deprived. Yum!

Serves: 4
Time: 25 mins
- Calories: 422
- Net carbs: 14g
- Protein: 48g
- Fat: 18g

Ingredients:
- 4 boneless, skinless chicken breasts of equal size
- 2 tablespoons minced garlic or garlic paste
- Salt and pepper, to taste
- 1 tablespoon dried oregano, divided
- Extra virgin olive oil
- 1/2 cup dry white wine
- Juice of 1 large lemon
- 1/2 cup chicken broth
- 1 cup finely chopped red onion
- 1 1/2 cup small-diced tomatoes
- 1/4 cup sliced green olives

To serve...
- Handful of fresh parsley, stems removed, chopped
- Feta cheese, crumbled

Method:
1. Make three small cuts into the chicken breasts and spread with the garlic, making sure some of the garlic goes into the guts.
2. Season with the salt, pepper and ½ the oregano.
3. Meanwhile, place a skillet over a medium heat and add the oil.
4. Add the chicken and cook until browned, turning as required.
5. Pour in the white wine and allow it to reduce to half, scraping away any burnt bits with a wooden spoon.
6. Add the lemon juice, broth and oregano, stir well then cover and cook for 15 minutes, turning the chicken halfway through.
7. Remove the lid then top with the onions, tomatoes and olives.
8. Cover again and cook for a further 5 minutes.
9. Remove the lid and add the parsley and feta cheese.
10. Serve and enjoy!

Chicken Pasta Bake

There's something so comforting about pasta bakes that they're my go-to whenever I feel in need of something warm and friendly in my tummy. When you give it a Mediterranean makeover, you can create a dish that's sin-free yet utterly amazing. Try it!

Serves: 5
Time: 1 hour 30 mins
- Calories: 829
- Net carbs: 83g
- Protein: 57g
- Fat: 29g

Ingredients:
For the chicken...
- 1 ½ lb. boneless, skinless chicken thighs, cut into bite-sized pieces
- 2 garlic cloves, thinly sliced
- 2-3 tablespoons marinade from artichoke hearts
- 4 sprigs of fresh oregano, leaves stripped
- Extra-virgin olive oil
- Red wine vinegar

For the bake...
- 1 lb. wholewheat Fusilli pasta
- 1 red onion, thinly sliced
- 1 pint grape or cherry tomatoes, whole
- ½ cup marinated artichoke hearts, roughly chopped
- ½ cup white beans, rinsed and drained
- ½ cup Kalamata olives, roughly chopped
- ⅓ cup parsley and basil leaves, roughly chopped
- 2-3 handfuls shredded mozzarella cheese
- Salt and pepper, to taste

To serve...
- Fresh parsley
- Fresh basil

Method:
1. Grab a large bowl and add the juice from the artichokes, garlic, oregano, and red wine vinegar. Stir well.
2. Add the chicken, stir again to coat then cover and place into the fridge to marinade for at least 30 minutes.
3. Preheat your oven to 425°F.
4. Take a casserole dish and add the onions and tomatoes. Drizzle with olive oil and seasonings.
5. Place into the oven and allow the tomatoes to soften and burst. This should take around 15 minutes.

6. Place a skillet over a medium heat and add a teaspoon of olive oil.
7. Remove the chicken from the marinade and cook in the pan, turning as needed.
8. Remove the casserole dish from the oven and add the pasta, chicken, artichokes, beans, olive and herbs. Stir well.
9. Sprinkle with grated cheese and pop back into the oven for about 5 minutes until the cheese melts.
10. Serve and enjoy.

Mozzarella Chicken Bake

Get the oven on! It's time to create a chicken bake that simply melts in your mouth and leaves you feeling like you've died and gone to heaven. Yes, it really IS that good.

Serves: 4
Time: 1 hour

- Calories: 693
- Net carbs: 3g
- Protein: 63g
- Fat: 45g

Ingredients:

- 4 boneless skinless chicken breasts
- 4 slices mozzarella cheese
- 1/2 cup mayonnaise
- 1/2 cup sour cream
- 3/4 cup grated parmesan cheese, divided
- 1/2 teaspoon salt
- 1/2 teaspoon pepper
- 1 teaspoon garlic powder

To serve…

- Cooked rice (opt)

Method:

1. Preheat the oven to 375°F and grease a 9"x 13" baking dish.
2. Place the chicken inside and top with the sliced cheese.
3. Take a medium bowl and add the mayonnaise, sour cream, ½ cup of the parmesan cheese, the salt, pepper and garlic powder. Stir well to combine.
4. Spread over the chicken and then sprinkle with the remaining parmesan.
5. Pop into the oven and bake for 1 hour.
6. Serve and enjoy.

Spiced Mediterranean Chicken

The addition of chili, coriander and paprika give this chicken dish an edge that you sometimes don't find in Mediterranean cooking, but you'll remember forever. Topped with Portuguese-style Piri-Piri sauce, you can make this blow your taste buds away (but feel free to skip if you're not a fan of spice).

Serves: 8
Time: 20 mins
- Calories: 153
- Net carbs: 7g
- Protein: 12g
- Fat: 8g

Ingredients:
- 2 tablespoons olive oil
- 2 lb. chicken thighs, skinless and boneless
- 2 cups white onion, chopped
- 1 teaspoon smoked paprika
- 1 teaspoon onion powder
- ¼ teaspoon chili pepper
- ½ teaspoon ground coriander seed
- 2 teaspoons dried parsley
- 2 teaspoons dried oregano
- Salt and black pepper, to taste
- 1 x 28 oz. can chopped tomato
- ½ cup black olives

Method:
1. Preheat your oven to 400°F.
2. Place a medium pan over a medium heat and add the olive oil.
3. Throw in the chicken and cook until browned then pop to one side.
4. Add the onions and cook for five minutes until soft.
5. Throw in the spices, salt, pepper and diced tomatoes and cook for another five minutes.
6. Pop the chicken back into the pot stir well then pop into the oven.
7. Cook for 15-30 minutes, until cooked through.
8. Serve and enjoy.

One Pot Greek Chicken & Lemon Rice

Somehow, the Greeks really know how to make rice dishes taste awesome. When you spoil your chicken with lemon and more oregano, you might find you want to eat this dish every single night. You have been warned!

Serves: 5
Time: 1 hour
- Calories: 667
- Net carbs: 33g
- Protein: 76g
- Fat: 23g

Ingredients:
- 2 lb. chicken thighs, skin on, bone in

For the marinade...
- Zest of one lemon
- 4 tablespoons fresh lemon juice
- 1 tablespoon dried oregano
- 4 garlic cloves, minced
- 1/2 teaspoon salt

For the rice...
- 1 1/2 tablespoon olive oil, divided
- 1 small onion, finely diced
- 1 cup long grain rice (brown if you can, but adjust cooking times accordingly)
- 1 1/2 cups chicken broth / stock
- 3/4 cup water
- 1 tablespoon dried oregano
- 3/4 teaspoon salt
- Black pepper

To serve...
- Finely chopped parsley or oregano (opt)
- Fresh lemon zest (opt)

Method:
1. Grab a large bowl and add the marinade ingredients. Stir well then add the chicken.
2. Stir to coat then cover and pop into the fridge for at least 30 minutes, preferably overnight.
3. Preheat the oven to 350°F.
4. Place a skillet over a medium heat and add ½ tablespoon of oil.
5. Remove the chicken from the marinade and fry until brown, flipping when needed.
6. Transfer the chicken onto an ovenproof dish then pop to one side.
7. Add the remaining oil to the skillet and add the onion. Cook for five minutes until soft.
8. Add the rice, broth, water, oregano, seasoning and reserved marinade and stir well.
9. Cover and cook for 20-30 minutes until the rice has absorbed all the water.

10. Open the lid, place the chicken on top and then cover.
11. Pop into the oven for 35 minutes until the chicken is cooked and the rice has absorbed all the water (add more liquid if needed.)
12. Serve and enjoy.

Harissa Chicken with Garbanzo Beans and Sweet Potatoes

I love roasted chicken and vegetable dishes like these because they're so simple to prepare, so healthy and you can throw the ingredients into your oven and practically forget them until it's time to tuck in. Serve with the yoghurt or herbs, or grab some tzatziki from your fridge and throw in on top. Wow!

Serves: 6
Time: 55 mins
- Calories: 398
- Net carbs: 36g
- Protein: 27g
- Fat: 26g

Ingredients:
- 1 1/2 lb. boneless chicken breasts or thighs
- 1/4 cup olive oil plus, more for drizzling
- Zest and juice of 1 lemon
- 1 lemon, sliced
- 2 tablespoons Harissa seasoning
- 1 tablespoon honey
- Salt and pepper, to taste
- 2 medium sweet potatoes, cut into 1" chunks
- 1 sweet onion, sliced
- 1 x 14 oz. garbanzo beans, drained
- 1/2 cup crumbled feta
- 1/3 cup green olives, smashed

To serve...
- Plain Greek yogurt
- Fresh mint or cilantro

Method:
1. Preheat the oven to 425°F and grease a baking sheet.
2. Find a large bowl and combine the chicken, olive oil, lemon juice and zest, harissa, honey and the salt and pepper. Toss to coat.
3. Add the sweet potatoes, onions and chickpeas, stir well, season and transfer to the baking tray.
4. Top with the lemon slices and pop into the oven for 45 minutes, turning halfway through.
5. Whilst it's cooking, take a small bowl and combine the feta, olives and a drizzle of olive oil.
6. Remove the chicken from the oven and serve with the feta and olive salad.

Seafood

Linguine and Zucchini Noodles with Shrimp

It's difficult to know why this dish tastes so good. Is it the tender and healthy zucchini? The filling and wholesome pasta? The delicious shrimp and equally tasty sauce? Who knows! Try it and decide for yourself.

Serves: 8
Time: 25 mins
- Calories: 531
- Net carbs: 52g
- Protein: 23g
- Fat: 28g

Ingredients:
- 1 lb. large shrimp, deveined and tails removed
- 1/3 cup plus 2 tablespoons extra virgin olive oil
- 4 large cloves garlic, minced
- Salt and pepper, to taste
- 3 medium size zucchinis, spiralized
- 1 x 12 oz. package whole wheat linguine
- 3 tablespoons butter
- Juice and zest of 1 lemon
- 1 teaspoon red chili flakes
- 1/2 cup grated parmesan cheese

To serve…
- Fresh chopped Italian parsley

Method:
1. Find a medium bowl and add the shrimp.
2. Add one tablespoon olive oil and two cloves of garlic, stir well, season then pop to one side.
3. Place a large pan over water over a medium heat and bring to the boil.
4. Add a pinch of salt then cook the linguine according to the directions on the package until al dente.
5. Remove the linguine from the pot and pop to one side, retaining the pasta water.
6. Next take a large pan, add one tablespoon of oil and pop over a medium heat.
7. Add the shrimp and cook for 5 minutes, turning as needed. Pop onto a plate.
8. Add the butter and remaining oil to the pan and cook the remaining garlic, lemon zest, lemon juice, red pepper flakes, and ½ cup reserved pasta water.
9. Cook for a minute, stirring often.
10. Add the zucchini to the pan and cook for a further minute then transfer to the pan that you used to cook the shrimp. Stir well to coat with the olive oil.
11. Add the linguine noodles and half of the parmesan cheese and stir
12. Add more pasta water if required then add the shrimp and zucchini, season again then stir.
13. Serve topped with the remaining parmesan and enjoy.

Shrimp Pasta with Roasted Red Peppers and Artichokes

This shrimp pasta is incredibly creamy, delicious and utterly moreish. And you know what? You're allowed to eat every bite on the Mediterranean diet! There's something about the combination of shrimp with feta that lights up my taste buds. Wow!

Serves: 8
Time: 35 mins
- Calories: 528
- Net carbs: 42g
- Protein: 32g
- Fat: 23g

Ingredients:
- 12 oz. pasta shapes, cooked
- 1 1/2 lb. medium shrimp, deveined
- 1/4 cup butter
- 3 cloves garlic, minced
- 1 x 12 oz. jar roasted red bell peppers, drained and chopped
- 1 cup canned artichoke hearts in water or brine, quartered
- 1/2 cup dry white wine
- 3 tablespoons drained capers
- 1/2 cup whipping cream
- 1 teaspoon finely shredded lemon zest
- 2 tablespoons lemon juice
- 3/4 cup crumbled feta cheese
- 2 oz. toasted pine nuts
- 1/4 cup snipped fresh basil

Method:
1. Place a skillet over a medium heat and add the butter.
2. Add the garlic and cook for a minute or two.
3. Add the shrimp and cook for 2 minutes, cooking often.
4. Throw in the peppers, artichokes, wine and capers. Stir well.
5. Bring to the boil then reduce the heat and simmer for 2 minutes until the shrimp are opaque.
6. Pour in the cream, plus the zest and juice. Stir well then reduce the heat.
7. Simmer for a further minute then remove from the heat.
8. Grab a large bowl and add the pasta, then pour in the sauce.
9. Stir and serve and enjoy with feta cheese, pine nuts and basil.

Baked Shrimp and Veggies

When you need a healthy dinner ready and on the table fast, choose this mouth-watering shrimp dish. With a light sauce made from olive oil and vinegar plus just the right amount of spice, it's healthy, tender and ready in under 30 minutes. What more could you want?

Serves: 4-6
Time: 25 mins
- Calories: 215
- Net carbs: 9g
- Protein: 21g
- Fat: 15g

Ingredients:
- 1 lb. asparagus, tough parts removed, cut into 2-inch pieces
- 2 cups cherry tomatoes
- 1 red onion, halved and thickly sliced
- 1 lb. large shrimp, peeled and deveined
- Extra-virgin olive oil
- Juice of ½ lemon
- Fresh chopped parsley for garnish

For the sauce...
- 1/3 cup extra virgin olive oil
- 1/4 cup white wine vinegar
- 1 teaspoon fresh grated ginger
- 1 teaspoon ground sumac
- 1 teaspoon ground cumin
- 1 teaspoon salt
- 1/2 teaspoon garlic powder
- 1/2 teaspoon ground black pepper

Method:
1. Preheat the oven 400°F and grease a large baking sheet.
2. Take a medium bowl and add the ingredients for the sauce. Stir well to combine.
3. Take a large bowl and add the veggies, then pour over ¼ of the sauce. Stir well to combine.
4. Place the veggies onto the baking sheet and spread out.
5. Pop into the oven to cook for 10 minutes.
6. Find a large bowl and add the shrimp then pour the remaining sauce over the top and stir.
7. Take the veggies from the oven then use a spoon to push them to one side of the baking sheet. Place the shrimp onto the other side, spreading out well.
8. Pop back into the oven for another five minutes until cooked.
9. Serve and enjoy.

Easy Baked Octopus

Back off now if you're scared of seafood that actually looks like seafood. Jump ahead to the next recipe. But if you want an octopus dish that is astonishingly good and you're worth waiting to get it just right, give this recipe a try.

Serves: 4-6
Time: 1 hour 45 mins
- Calories: 289
- Net carbs: 4g
- Protein: 45g
- Fat: 9g

Ingredients:
- 2 ½- 3 lb. octopus, fresh
- 2 tablespoons balsamic vinegar
- 3 tablespoons olive oil
- Pinch of pepper
- 2 bay leaves
- 5 allspice kernels
- 1/2 teaspoon oregano

To serve...
- Extra olive oil
- Balsamic vinegar

Method:
1. Preheat the oven to 320°F.
2. Place the octopus onto a flat surface, clean well and remove its tooth.
3. Pop two sheets of foil onto your counter then add a piece of baking paper to the middle.
4. Place the octopus into the middle and drizzle with the olive oil and balsamic vinegar.
5. Season with the remaining ingredients then fold up in the baking paper and foil.
6. Place onto a baking tray and cook for 1 ½ hours until tender.
7. Remove from the foil then serve and enjoy.

Saucy Greek Baked Shrimp

Nothing beats the smell of this delicious Greek dish when it comes out of the oven. It's mouth-wateringly good. Allspice, cinnamon and dill are an unexpected combo that add a softer and more fragrant edge to the dish and help balance the garlic and feta. Yum!

Serves: 4
Time: 35 mins
- Calories: 285
- Net carbs: 7g
- Protein: 27g
- Fat: 16g

Ingredients:
- 1 lb. large peeled and deveined shrimp
- 1/2 teaspoon red pepper flakes
- 1/4 teaspoon salt
- 3 tablespoons olive oil
- 1 medium onion, chopped
- 3 garlic cloves, minced
- 1 x 15 oz. can crushed tomatoes
- 1/2 teaspoon ground allspice
- 1/2 teaspoon ground cinnamon
- 1/2 cup crumbled feta cheese
- 2 tablespoons chopped fresh dill

Method:
1. Preheat the oven to 375°F.
2. Grab a medium bowl and add the red pepper flakes and salt. Stir well then pop to one side.
3. Place a skillet over a medium heat and add the oil.
4. Add the onion and garlic and cook for five minutes until soft.
5. Add the spices and stir well. Cook for about 30 seconds.
6. Throw in the tomatoes and simmer for 20 minutes.
7. Remove from the heat then add the shrimp.
8. Add the feta cheese and pop into the oven for 15-20 minutes until the cheese has melted.
9. Sprinkle with the fresh dill then serve and enjoy.

Italian Seafood Stew

With a hearty base of tomatoes, pepper, onion and garlic, as much seafood as you can possibly fit in and plenty of surprises, this Italian Seafood Stew is easy, relatively fast and perfect for sharing with a happy crowd.

Serves: 8
Time: 45 mins

- Calories: 961
- Net carbs: 34g
- Protein: 47g
- Fat: 80g

Ingredients:

- 2 cloves garlic, chopped
- 1 onion, chopped
- ½ red pepper, chopped
- 1 ½ cups chopped tomatoes
- 3 ½ oz. squid, cut into squares
- 1 halibut fillet, cut into 6 pieces
- 10 jumbo shrimp
- 8 fresh mussels
- 1 teaspoon thyme
- 1 teaspoon smoked paprika
- 1 pinch saffron
- ½ teaspoon white sugar
- 1 ½ cups fish broth
- ¼ cup water
- 10 blanched almonds, dry roasted
- 4 tablespoons extra virgin olive oil
- Salt and pepper, to taste

To serve...

- Fresh parsley, chopped

Method:

1. Place a large skillet over a medium heat and add the oil.
2. Season the squid with salt and add to the pan. Cook for 2 minutes then remove from the pan and pop to one side.
3. Add the onion, red pepper and garlic and cook for 5 minutes until soft.
4. Add the herbs and spices and stir well.
5. Throw in the tomato, sugar and salt and stir well. Cook for five minutes.
6. Add the fish broth, water and saffron, stir well then bring to the boil.
7. Reduce to a simmer.
8. Grab a pestle and mortar and add the almonds, 2 tablespoons of fresh parsley and 1 tablespoon of olive oil. Grind to a paste.
9. Add the almond mixture to the pan of tomato sauce and stir well.
10. Add the halibut, squid, shrimp and mussels, stir well and cover the pan.
11. Cook for five minutes then serve and enjoy.

Fish

Baked Fish with Artichokes and Olives

Artichokes and olives come together to make this delicious dish, perfect for a midweek meal when you want something tasty on the table but you honestly don't have the time. Feel free to add your favorite veggies to make it even more amazing.

Serves: 4
Time: 35 mins
- Calories: 417
- Net carbs: 20g
- Protein: 29g
- Fat: 25g

Ingredients:
- 1 ½ tablespoons olive oil
- 1/2 yellow onion, chopped
- 6 cloves garlic
- 2 x 14 oz. cans chopped tomatoes, liquid drained
- 1/4 cup fresh chopped basil, packed
- Salt and pepper, to taste
- 4 cod fillets
- 1/2 cup feta cheese, crumbled
- 15 oz. artichoke hearts, liquid drained
- 2 Roma tomatoes, roughly chopped
- 4 oz. kalamata olives
- 2 tablespoons capers
- 1 lemon, sliced

To serve...
- Feta cheese
- Basil
- Capers

Method:
1. Preheat the oven to 375°F.
2. Place an oven-proof skillet over a medium heat and add the oil.
3. Cook the onion and garlic for 5 minutes until soft.
4. Add the tomatoes, basil, salt and pepper and stir to combine.
5. Bring to the boil then remove from the hat.
6. Lay the fish on top, sprinkle with cheese, place the artichokes, tomato slices and lemon slices over the top.
7. Crown with olives and capers then pop into the oven.
8. Bake for 15-25 minutes until cooked.
9. Serve and enjoy!

Salmon with Paprika and Fennel

Salmon, dill, paprika, fennel and lemon...What more do you need for a delicious meal?

Serves: 2
Time: 45 mins
- Calories: 372
- Net carbs: 4g
- Protein: 22g
- Fat: 30g

Ingredients:
- 2 x 6 oz. salmon fillets, skin on
- Salt and pepper, to taste
- 1 teaspoon smoked paprika
- ½ teaspoon fennel seeds, lightly crushed
- 1 lemon, zested then halved
- ¼ cup fresh chopped dill
- 3 tablespoons extra-virgin olive oil

Method:
1. Place the salmon onto a flat surface and season with the salt and pepper, ½ teaspoon paprika, ¼ teaspoon fennel seeds, half the lemon zest and half of the dill.
2. Squeeze the juice of half a lemon over each piece.
3. Place a skillet over a very low heat and add the oil.
4. Cook the salmon for 20-25 minutes until perfect.
5. Serve and enjoy.

Striped Bass with Provencal Tomatoes

This incredibly healthy fish dish is tender, rich and perfect for a romantic meal, a family dinner or any other kind of gathering your heart desires. It's another dish that's ready and on the table fast. Enjoy!

Serves: 4
Time: 20 mins
- Calories: 364
- Net carbs: 17g
- Protein: 45g
- Fat: 16g

Ingredients:
- 4 x 6 oz. striped bass fillets, skin on
- Salt, to taste
- Herbs de Provence, to taste
- 1 tablespoon Dijon mustard
- 3 medium heirloom tomatoes, diced
- 1/3 cup mixed pitted olives
- 1 tablespoon capers
- 1 clove garlic minced
- 2 tablespoons olive oil
- 1 tablespoon white wine vinegar

To serve...
- Fresh parsley, thyme, or chives

Method:
1. Preheat the broiler and grease a baking sheet.
2. Place the fish fillets onto the baking sheet and season with salt and herbs.
3. Cover the tops with the mustard.
4. Take a medium bowl and add the tomatoes, olives, capers, garlic, olive oil, vinegar and ½ teaspoon salt. Stir well to combine.
5. Spoon the tomato mixture over the fish then place under the broiler for around 10 minutes, turning halfway through cooking.
6. Sprinkle the fresh herbs over the top then serve and enjoy.

Tuna Couscous with Pepperoncini

Anyone in the mood for some spice? Then create this easy North African inspired dish for a well-balanced and satisfying dish that is perfect as a light dinner and wonderful for lunch too.

Serves: 4
Time: 15 mins
- Calories: 289
- Net carbs: 46g
- Protein: 14g
- Fat: 6g

Ingredients:

For the couscous...
- 1 cup chicken broth or water
- 1¼ cups couscous
- ¾ teaspoon salt

For the salad...
- 2 x 5 oz. cans oil packed tuna
- 1 pint cherry tomatoes, halved
- ½ cup sliced pepperoncini
- ⅓ cup chopped fresh parsley
- ¼ cup capers

To serve...
- Extra-virgin olive oil
- Salt and pepper, to taste
- 1 lemon, quartered

Method:
1. Make the couscous according to the instructions on the packet.
2. Take a medium bowl and add the tuna, tomatoes, pepperoncini, parsley and capers. Stir well to combine.
3. Fluff the couscous with a fork, season well and drizzle with olive oil.
4. Add the tuna mixture to the top and serve and enjoy.

Parmesan Pesto Tilapia

You can't go wrong when it comes to a crunchy cheesy topping with herby and satisfying pesto and as many tomatoes as you can fit onto the plate. This one is perfect when served with a big salad, a huge chunk of bread and a glass of wine.

Serves: 4
Time: 15 mins
- Calories: 680
- Net carbs: 8g
- Protein: 98g
- Fat: 28g

Ingredients:
- 4 x 6 oz. tilapia filets
- 1/4 cup basil pesto
- 1/2 cup freshly grated parmesan cheese
- 1 cup fresh chopped tomatoes
- Salt and pepper, to taste

To serve...
- Lemon juice, to taste
- Melted butter, to taste

Method:
1. Preheat your broiler and grease a baking sheet.
2. Place the fish onto the baking tray, sprinkle each fillet with 2 tablespoons of cheese then pop under the broiler for 10 minutes.
3. Remove from the broiler and top each fillet with a tablespoon of pesto and the fresh tomato. Sprinkle with extra parmesan then pop back under the broiler for a minute or two.
4. Serve and enjoy with the butter and fresh lemon.

Rosemary Citrus One Pan Baked Salmon

Salmon is a great source of omega-3 fatty acids which help feed your brain and nervous system, boost your mood, and help you look and feel amazing. Cooked with the uplifting citrus flavors of lemon and orange, your taste buds will be lifted to the heavens, and you'll feel utterly spoiled.

Serves: 3
Time: 20 mins
- Calories: 345
- Net carbs: 7g
- Protein: 25g
- Fat: 22g

Ingredients:
- 1/3 cup olive oil
- Salt and pepper, to taste
- 2 tablespoons fresh orange juice
- 2 tablespoon fresh rosemary, plus 1-2 extra sprigs to garnish
- 1 tablespoon lemon juice
- 1/2 teaspoon garlic, minced
- 1/4 teaspoon grated dried orange zest, divided
- 1 bunch thin asparagus, trimmed
- Olive oil or melted butter, to drizzle
- 10–12 oz. salmon

To serve...
- Thinly sliced orange
- Lemon rind
- 1/4 teaspoon lemon pepper (opt.)

Method:
1. Preheat the oven to 400°F and grease a baking dish.
2. Grab a medium bowl and add the orange juice, lemon, rosemary, olive oil, salt, pepper, ¼ teaspoon orange zest and garlic. Stir well then pop to one side.
3. Place the asparagus into the baking dish and drizzle with olive oil.
4. Add a pinch of pepper seasoning then place the salmon between the spears, skin down.
5. Drizzle with the marinade and add the slices of lemon on top of the salmon.
6. Top with the sprigs of rosemary plus extra lemon peel and seasonings
7. Pop into the oven for 10-15 minutes until cooked to perfection.
8. Serve and enjoy.

Pan-Fried Cod with Orange and Swiss Chard

More orange here, but this time combined with the bitter flavors of Swiss Chard, sweet red onion and plenty of parsley to make a fast meal you'll never forget.

Serves: 4
Time: 30 mins

- Calories: 296
- Net carbs: 35g
- Protein: 7g
- Fat: 16g

Ingredients:

- 4 x 6 oz. cod fillets
- Salt and black pepper, to taste
- 1 cup all-purpose flour
- ½ teaspoon cayenne pepper
- 4 tablespoons extra-virgin olive oil
- 1 red onion, thinly sliced
- 1 orange, halved and thinly sliced
- ¼ cup chopped fresh parsley, plus more for garnish
- 2½ cups chopped Swiss chard
- Orange wedges, for serving

Method:

1. Place the cod fillets onto a plate and season well.
2. Grab a large bowl and add the flour and cayenne pepper. Stir well to combine
3. Place the cod into the flour and pat to coat well.
4. Place a medium pan over a medium heat and add the olive oil.
5. Add the cod and pan-fry for about 5-10 minutes until browned and cook on both sides.
6. Remove the cod from the pan and drain most of the oil.
7. Add the onion and orange and cook for five minutes, until the onion is tender.
8. Stir through the chard and the parsley and cook for 3-4 minutes.
9. Serve and enjoy.

Pan-Seared Cod with Pomegranate Salsa

I love the simplicity of the cod and the sweet complexity of the homemade spicy onion-chili-pomegranate salsa. There's something so satisfying about biting into those pomegranate gems and allowing the combined spice and juice to envelope your mouth...

Serves: 4
Time: 20 mins

- Calories: 111
- Net carbs: 13g
- Protein: 6g
- Fat: 5g

Ingredients:

For the fish...

- 4 filets cod or halibut
- 1/2 teaspoon garlic powder
- Salt and pepper, to taste
- 1 tablespoon olive oil or butter

For the pomegranate salsa...

- 1 cup fresh pomegranate
- 1/3 cup finely chopped fresh cilantro
- 1/4 cup finely chopped red onion
- 1 jalapeno, cored and finely chopped
- Juice of one lime
- Pinch ground cumin
- Salt and pepper, to taste

For the kale...

- Fresh kale, to taste
- 1 garlic clove, sliced
- Olive oil

Method:

1. Place the fish onto a flat surface and season with the cumin, salt and pepper.
2. Place a skillet over a medium heat and add the oil.
3. Add the fish and cook for 5-10 minutes until browned, flipping halfway through cooking.
4. Meanwhile, grab a large bowl and add the ingredients for the salsa and stir well to combine.
5. Place the fish onto a plate then top with the salsa.
6. Add a drop more olive oil to the pan and add the garlic. Cook for a minute or two then throw in the kale and stir until cooked.
7. Serve with the fish then enjoy!

Honey-Mustard Sheet Pan Salmon

I've lost count of the number of times I've been begged for the secret ingredient in this recipe, but honestly, there isn't one. With just the right combo of honey and mustard, a premium salmon fillet and plenty of fresh veggies, there's no way you could ever go wrong.

Serves: 5
Time: 45 mins
- Calories: 247
- Net carbs: 24g
- Protein: 15g
- Fat: 11g

Ingredients:
For the marinade...
- 1 tablespoon raw honey
- 1 tablespoon coarse-grain mustard
- ½ teaspoon white wine vinegar
- ½ teaspoon oregano
- Salt and pepper, to taste

For the salmon...
- 2 lb. salmon fillet, pin bones removed

For the veggies...
- 2 ½ cups peeled, seeded, and cubed butternut squash
- 12 oz. Brussels sprouts, trimmed and halved
- 2 cups cherry tomatoes
- 2 tablespoons olive oil
- ½ teaspoon freshly squeezed lemon juice
- ¼ teaspoon garlic powder
- ¼ teaspoon onion powder
- ¼ teaspoon dried oregano, divided
- ⅛ teaspoon ground turmeric
- 1 lemon, thinly sliced crosswise

Method:
1. Preheat the oven to 400°F and grease a baking dish and a baking sheet.
2. Grab a small bowl and add the ingredients for the marinade. Stir well to combine.
3. Place the salmon into the baking dish and pour the marinade over the top.
4. Pop into the fridge for 30 minutes to marinade.
5. Take a large bowl and add all the ingredients for the veggies. Stir well to combine.
6. Place onto the baking sheet, spreading it out well.
7. Remove the salmon from the fridge, allow any excess marinade to drip away then place onto the veggies.
8. Top with lemon slices then pop into the oven for 15-20 minutes until perfectly cooked.

Fish Puttanesca en Papillote

I have to say that I'd never tried halibut which tasted quite as moist and tender as this one. Gently baking in paper and seasoned with capers, olive and tomatoes, it's certainly a dish to remember. If you want to be even more authentic, feel free to add anchovies and extra olives.

Serves: 2-3
Time: 30 mins
- Calories: 248
- Net carbs: 18g
- Protein: 21g
- Fat: 14g

Ingredients:
- 2 x 6-8 oz. halibut fillets
- 8 oz. green beans
- 2 cloves garlic, minced
- 2 tablespoons extra virgin olive oil
- Salt and pepper, to taste
- 4 tablespoons marinara sauce
- 1 lemon, ½ for serving, half sliced into several thin slices
- 2 teaspoons capers, drained
- 2 tablespoons kalamata olives, halved
- 1 teaspoon fresh oregano leaves
- 1/4 teaspoon crushed red pepper flakes (opt)
- 2 tablespoons fresh basil, cut into thin ribbons

Method:
1. Preheat the oven to 400°F and line a baking sheet with two sheets of parchment paper.
2. Place the haricot verts into the middle and place the fish over the top.
3. Pop the garlic, olive oil, salt, pepper and marinara sauce over the top.
4. Place lemon slices over each fillet and scatter the capers and the olives over the top.
5. Sprinkle with oregano and crushed red pepper then fold the paper over, creating a package with the fish.
6. Place the baking sheet with the fish into the oven and cook for 18-22 minutes, checking often.
7. Serve with fresh basil and lemon juice. Enjoy!

Hemp and Walnut Crusted Salmon with Broccoli and Kimchi Cauliflower Rice

Give your salmon a makeover with this crunchy hemp and walnut crusted dish. Simple and utterly delicious, it tastes best served with whatever green leafy veggies you have on hand plus plenty of tomatoes. Of course, the Kimchi isn't Mediterranean, but it certainly adds an awesome kick and it's great for your gut. Try it!

Serves: 2
Time: 30 mins
- Calories: 720
- Net carbs: 50g
- Protein: 33g
- Fat: 46g

Ingredients:
- 10 walnuts, finely chopped
- 2 tablespoons hemp seeds
- Salt and pepper, to taste
- 1 lemon, halved
- Extra-virgin olive oil
- 2 x 6 oz. wild salmon
- 2 tablespoons olive oil, divided
- 1 head broccoli, sliced into florets
- 1 small head of cauliflower, riced
- 1 cup kimchi, roughly chopped

Method:
1. Preheat the oven to 275°F and place a sheet of parchment paper onto a baking sheet
2. Grab a small bowl and add the walnuts, hemp seeds, salt and pepper. Stir well to combine.
3. Place the salmon onto the parchment paper and drizzle with olive oil and squeeze the lemon juice over the top.
4. Sprinkle the nut mixture over the top and press into the fish.
5. Pop into the oven and cook for 15-30 minutes until cooked to taste.
6. Place a skillet over a medium heat and add 1 tablespoon of olive oil.
7. Throw in the broccoli and cook for 10 minutes, stirring often.
8. Remove from the pan and place into a bowl. Season well and squeeze with more lemon juice.
9. Place more olive oil into the skillet and add the cauliflower. Cook for 10 minutes until brown.
10. Add the kimchi and cook for 3 minutes more.
11. Place the kimchi cauliflower onto a serving dish, scatter with the broccoli and place the salmon over the top.
12. Serve and enjoy.

Spiced Moroccan Halibut

Take a trip to African with this spiced fish dish. Featuring spices like paprika, cinnamon, turmeric, red pepper flakes and cayenne, you can feel like you're taking a walk through a colorful spice market whilst enjoying the summertime flavors of zucchini, onions, carrots and garlic.

Serves: 4
Time: 20 mins
- Calories: 209
- Net carbs: 11g
- Protein: 26g
- Fat: 6g

Ingredients:
- 1 tablespoon extra-virgin olive oil
- 1 zucchini, finely chopped
- 1 onion, finely chopped
- 2 large carrots, finely chopped
- 1 clove garlic, crushed and minced
- 1 x 15oz. can whole tomatoes
- 2 teaspoons paprika
- 1/4 teaspoon turmeric
- 1/2 teaspoon cinnamon
- 1/4 teaspoon cayenne pepper
- 1 teaspoon Himalayan sea salt
- Dash freshly ground pepper
- 1/2 teaspoon red pepper flakes
- 2 tablespoon capers
- 1 lb. halibut

Method:
1. Place a skillet over a medium heat and add the oil.
2. Throw in the garlic and cook for a minute, then add the zucchini, onion and carrots. Cook until the veggies are soft.
3. Add the tomatoes, paprika, turmeric, cinnamon, cayenne, salt, pepper and red pepper flakes. Stir well to combine.
4. Bring to the boil then turn down the heat and simmer for five minutes.
5. Place the fish into the sauce, spoon the sauce over the top until it's completely submerged then cover and cook for 7-10 minutes.
6. Add the capers then serve and enjoy.

Sicilian Style Salmon with Garlic Broccoli and Tomatoes

The Sicilians really know how to transform a simple piece of fish into something that melts in your mouth and leaves you craving more. When you try this Italian dish, you'll never want to eat deep-fried fish again, trust me.

Serves: 4
Time: 25 mins
- Calories: 303
- Net carbs: 15g
- Protein: 39g
- Fat: 35g

Ingredients:
- 4 salmon fillets
- Extra virgin olive oil
- Juice and zest of 1 lemon
- 1 teaspoon red pepper flakes
- 1 teaspoon paprika
- Salt and pepper, to taste
- 1 large head of broccoli, cut into florets
- 1 cup cherry tomatoes
- 2 cloves garlic, minced or grated
- 2 tablespoons chopped fresh oregano
- Splash of white wine
- 1/2 cup pitted kalamata olives

Method:
1. Place a skillet over a medium heat and add the olive oil.
2. Pop the salmon onto a flat surface and drizzle with olive oil and lemon juice.
3. Sprinkle with the chili flakes, paprika, salt and pepper.
4. Transfer to the skillet and cook for about 3 minutes on each side until starting to brown.
5. Remove from the pan and pop to one side.
6. Add extra oil to the pan if needed then add the broccoli and cook for five minutes until soft.
7. Throw in the tomatoes, garlic, oregano and lemon zest, season well then cook for 5 minutes.
8. Add the wine and stir well to form a sauce.
9. Throw in the olives, add the salmon and warm through.
10. Serve and enjoy.

Sardines with Fennel and Orange

Sardines are rich and delicious and when teamed with fennel, garlic and orange, they somehow transform into a healthy and nourishing meal that is simply out of this world. Serve with a simple salad.

Serves: 2-4
Time: 20 mins
- Calories: 309
- Net carbs: 10g
- Protein: 12g
- Fat: 23g

Ingredients:
- 3 tablespoons extra-virgin olive oil
- 1 onion, thinly sliced
- 4 garlic cloves, thinly sliced
- 2 baby fennel bulbs, fronds reserved
- 1 teaspoon fennel seeds
- Zested rind of 1 orange
- 1 tablespoon orange juice
- 1 tablespoon Pernod
- 1 tablespoon white wine vinegar
- 12 whole sardines

For brushing...
- Olive oil
- 1 tablespoon lemon juice

Method:
1. Place a large skillet over a medium heat and add the oil.
2. Add the onion and garlic and cook for 5 minutes until soft.
3. Throw in the fennel and fennel seeds and cook for five minutes until soft.
4. Add the orange zest and juice, Pernod, and vinegar and turn the heat up to high.
5. Reduce down until thick and syrupy, season to taste then pop to one side.
6. Place a grill pan over a medium heat.
7. Brush the sardines with olive oil, season well and place into the grill pan for 5-6 minutes, turning halfway through cooking.
8. Place the fennel and orange onto a serving plate and top with the salmon.
9. Serve and enjoy.

Sardine and Chili Fettuccine with Pine Nuts and Lemon

Why didn't anyone tell me how good sardines and fettuccine tasted together? I've wasted my life eating lesser-tasting pasta dishes when I could have been feasting on this stuff. That's why I've decided to share the secret and save you years of your life. You're welcome.

Serves: 4-6
Time: 15 mins

- Calories: 564
- Net carbs: 40g
- Protein: 38g
- Fat: 29g

Ingredients:

- 1/3 cup olive oil
- 2 ½ oz. pine nuts
- ½ cup each coarsely chopped flat-leaf parsley and oregano
- 2 garlic cloves, thinly sliced
- 1 long red chili, thinly sliced
- 12 marinated butterflied sardines, coarsely torn
- Juice and zest of 2 lemons
- 14 oz. dried wholemeal fettuccine

Method:

1. Place a saucepan over a medium heat and add half the oil.
2. Add the pine nuts and cook for 2-3 minutes until golden.
3. Remove from the oil then pop into a bowl. Add the herbs and stir well to combine.
4. Place the remaining oil into a medium skillet and pop over a medium heat.
5. Add the garlic and chili and cook for a minute until fragrant.
6. Throw in the sardines and stir well to warm. Remove from the heat.
7. Add the lemon zest, juice, half the pine nut mixture and seasoning. Stir well to combine.
8. Meanwhile, cook the pasta according to the cooking instructions on the packet.
9. Drain the pasta and return to the pan.
10. Add the sardine mixture then stir well to combine, breaking up the fish slightly.
11. Serve and enjoy.

Vegetarian & Vegan

Vegan Moussaka

Perfect for sharing and awesome for parties, this luscious vegan moussaka combines the traditional Mediterranean elements from the original recipe and creates a stunningly tasty vegan version. Tasting miles better than the original, it combines green lentils, eggplant and zucchini, bathes it in a tomato-garlic sauce and tops it all off with delicious potato slices. Yes, it does take time but it's very much worth it.

Serves: 12
Time: 1-2 hours
- Calories: 274
- Net carbs: 34g
- Protein: 7g
- Fat: 8g

Ingredients:
- 3 ½ lb. large russet potatoes, peeled and cut into chunks
- 4 cloves garlic, peeled
- 1/4 cup plus 2 tablespoon olive oil, divided
- 1 large onion, chopped
- 3 tablespoons dried oregano
- 2 x 15 oz. cans chopped tomatoes
- 2/3 cup green lentils
- 1 bay leaf
- 1 cinnamon stick
- 2 medium eggplants, sliced
- 2 small zucchinis, sliced
- 3 tomatoes, thinly sliced

Method:
1. Place a pan of water over a medium heat and bring to the boil.
2. Add the potatoes and garlic and cook for 10 minutes until soft.
3. Drain the potatoes but reserve the liquid until later.
4. Add the ¼ cup olive oil and 2 cups of the cooking liquid then mash with a fork or potato masher. Season well then pop to one side.
5. Place a pan over a medium heat, add the remaining olive oil and then cook the onion and oregano for five minutes until soft.
6. Throw in the tomatoes, lentils, bay leaf, cinnamon and 3 cups of the potato cooking liquid.
7. Cover, reduce the heat and cook for 45 minutes until the lentils are tender.
8. Remove the bay leaf and cinnamon and use an immersion blender to blend. Season then pop to one side.
9. Preheat the oven to 350°F and grease a 13" x 9" baking sheet.
10. Place about 1 ½ cups of the lentils into the bottom, then add a layer of eggplant, then zucchini and tomatoes.

11. Add 2 more cups of lentils then half of the potatoes over this.
12. Top with another layer of eggplant then another layer of lentils.
13. Top with potatoes then place into the oven.
14. Bake for 1 ½ hours until browned.

Stuffed Grape Leaves Casserole

This classic Greek recipe is much quicker and easier than it might look at first. Precook your rice and you'll have a head start that will demand just 30 minutes more for an epic veggie-friendly dinner.

Serves: 8
Time: 1 hour

- Calories: 341
- Net carbs: 42g
- Protein: 8g
- Fat: 15g

Ingredients:

- 30 jarred or fresh grape leaves
- 2 tablespoon olive oil
- 1 large onion, finely diced
- 1 cup brown rice
- 2 cups tomato juice or vegetable juice
- 1 cup chopped unsalted, hulled pistachios
- 1 cup chopped fresh parsley
- 1 cup chopped fresh mint
- 1 cup raisins or dried currants
- 1/4 cup lemon juice

To serve...

- 1 lemon, sliced, for garnish

Method:

1. Take a medium bowl, add some boiling water and submerge the grape leaves. Leave for two minutes to soften then drain and pop to one side.
2. Place a large saucepan over a medium heat, add the oil and then add the onion, cooking for 5 minutes until soft.
3. Add the rice and the water and bring to a boil.
4. Cover and cook for 20-30 minutes until the liquid has been absorbed.
5. Remove from the heat and add the tomato juice, pistachios, parsley, mint, raisins and lemon juice. Stir well to combine.
6. Preheat the oven to 350°F and grease a baking dish.
7. Carefully dry the grape leaves then line the baking dish with them, letting some leaves hang over the edges.
8. Spoon half of the rice mixture onto the rape leaves and spread well.
9. Top with more grape leaves then add another layer of rice.
10. Top with another layer of grape leaves and fold over the leaves at the edges to seal.
11. Brush with olive oil then bake for 30 minutes until brown.
12. Serve and enjoy.

Paella Primavera

Do you know what I love most about paella? It's the fact that you can throw pretty much anything you like into the dish and you'll have a filling and satisfying meal that ticks all the nutritional boxes and leaves you feeling good. This is my favorite combo. Enjoy!

Serves: 4-6
Time: 20 mins

- Calories: 211
- Net carbs: 35g
- Protein: 5g
- Fat: 3g

Ingredients:

- 2 1/2 teaspoons olive oil
- 1 red bell pepper, chopped
- 6 green onions, thinly sliced
- 3 cups vegetable broth
- 3 cloves garlic, minced
- 1 teaspoon crumbled saffron threads
- 1 cup short-grain white rice
- 3 cups broccoli florets
- 1 cup fresh or frozen baby peas
- 1 cup halved grape or cherry tomatoes
- 12 pitted green olives, halved
- 12 pitted black olives, halved
- 1 lemon, cut into wedges
- 1/4 cup chopped fresh parsley

Method:

1. Place a large skillet over a medium heat and add the oil.
2. Throw in the peppers and onions and cook for five minutes, stirring often.
3. Add the broth, garlic and saffron and bring to the boil.
4. Sprinkle with the rice then reduce the heat, cover and simmer for 10 minutes.
5. Remove the lid and the broccoli, peas, tomatoes and olives. Do not stir.
6. Cover and cook for a further 5-8 minutes until tender.
7. Remove from the heat and leave to rest for 5 minutes.
8. Season then serve and enjoy.

Portuguese Tomato Rice

This recipe came to me via a close Portuguese friend who claimed that it was fast, inexpensive to make and very delicious. And to be honest, I was skeptical. How could rice and tomatoes ever impress? But I'll admit that I was very wrong. The secret lies in the spice...

Serves: 4
Time: 40 mins
- Calories: 567
- Net carbs: 51g
- Protein: 12g
- Fat: 5g

Ingredients:
- 1 tablespoon olive oil
- 1 onion, diced
- 1 garlic clove, minced
- 1 teaspoon smoked paprika
- Pinch of cayenne chili pepper, to taste
- 1 cup long-grain rice (brown if you can, increase cooking time accordingly)
- 1 vegetable stock cube
- 2 1/2 cups water
- 3 tomatoes, peeled and diced
- 1 x 14 oz. can black beans, drained and rinsed
- Bunch of fresh cilantro, roughly chopped
- Salt and pepper, to taste

Method:
1. Grab a saucepan and place over a medium heat.
2. Add the oil then cook the onion and garlic for five minutes until soft.
3. Add the paprika and cayenne and fry for another couple of minutes.
4. Throw in the rice and fry again for about five minutes to allow the flavors to combine.
5. Add the stock, tomatoes, beans and water and stir to combine.
6. Cover and bring to the boil then turn down and cook for 10-15 minutes until soft.
7. Serve and enjoy.

Appetizers and Side Dishes
Greek Spinach and Rice

Classic spinach and rice is a dish that works brilliantly with any meal and can be on the table fast. It's also completely vegan and can be turned into an entire meal by itself if you throw in a can of your favorite beans.

Serves: 2-4
Time: 30 mins
- Calories: 165
- Net carbs: 23g
- Protein: 5g
- Fat: 5g

Ingredients:
- 1 lb. fresh spinach, rinsed
- Juice of half lemon
- 1 onion, chopped
- 2 ½ tablespoons olive oil plus more for drizzling
- 1 teaspoon dry mint
- 1-2 tablespoons chopped dill
- 2/3 cups water
- 1/3 cup medium grain rice
- Salt and pepper, to taste
- 1 tablespoon tomato paste (opt.)

Method:
1. Place a large pan over a medium heat and add a teaspoon of the olive oil, plus the lemon juice and spinach. Heat until the spinach starts to wilt then remove from the heat.
2. Take another pan, pop over a medium heat and add the remaining oil.
3. Cook the onion for around 5 minutes until soft.
4. Add the spinach, mint, dill and water then stir well and bring to the boil.
5. Add the rice, season well then simmer for around 20 minutes until the rice is soft.
6. Serve with lemon juice, olive oil and feta. Enjoy!

Greek Style Green Beans

Perfectly simple, perfectly delicious and perfectly right for your next meal. That's what this dish is. Wow!

Serves: 2-4
Time: 45 mins
- Calories: 558
- Net carbs: 18g
- Protein: 4g
- Fat: 54g

Ingredients:
- ½ cup olive oil
- 1 onion chopped
- 1 lb. green beans
- 1 medium potato, sliced in ¼" slices
- 1 x 14 oz. can chopped tomatoes
- ¼ cup chopped parsley
- 1 teaspoon sugar
- Salt and pepper, to taste

Method:
1. Take a medium pan, place over a medium heat and add the olive oil.
2. Add the onion and cook for five minutes until soft.
3. Throw in the potatoes and beans, stir well to coat with the olive oil and continue to cook for another 3-5 minutes.
4. Add the tomatoes, parsley, sugar, salt and pepper and stir well.
5. Add enough water to cover the beans then cover with the lid and simmer for 30 minutes.
6. Serve and enjoy.

Roasted Potatoes with Lemon and Garlic

I'm a big fan of roasted potatoes and I'll find any excuse to include them in my meals practically every day of the week. This is one of my favorite versions, flavored with lemon, garlic and a hit of allspice.

Serves: 6
Time: 1 hour 20 mins
- Calories: 724
- Net carbs: 27g
- Protein: 16g
- Fat: 63g

Ingredients:
- 2 lb. potatoes, cut in small wedges
- ½ cup olive oil
- 2-3 teaspoons dry oregano
- 1-2 tablespoons lemon juice
- 3 cloves garlic, chopped
- 3 allspice berries
- ½ teaspoon salt freshly ground pepper

Method:
1. Preheat the oven to 400°F and grab a large baking pan.
2. Grab a bowl and add the potatoes plus all the other ingredients (except the water).
3. Stir well to combine and transfer to the baking pan.
4. Add the water to the pan and allow to come about halfway up the potatoes.
5. Pop into the oven and roast for 10 minutes.
6. Reduce the heat to 320°F and continue to roast for 45 minutes more.
7. Serve and enjoy.

Herb Roasted Olives

Hold the popcorn! These roasted olives are the perfect healthy replacement. Garlic, oregano and just the right amount of seasoning are all it takes to make a snack that's perfect for sharing!

Makes: 1 cup
Time: 15 mins
- Calories: 364
- Net carbs: 7g
- Protein: 1g
- Fat: 34g

Ingredients:
- 1 cup olives
- 1 ½ tablespoon olive oil
- 1 clove garlic, minced
- 2 teaspoons oregano
- Salt and pepper, to taste
- Lemon zest
- Chopped parsley

Method:
1. Preheat your oven to 430°F and cover a baking sheet with foil.
2. Take a bowl and add all the ingredients, then stir well to combine
3. Season well then pop into the oven for 12 minutes.
4. Sprinkle with parsley and lemon peel then serve and enjoy.

Peach Bruschetta

I can almost guarantee that you've never tasted bruschetta quite as tasty as this one. Packed with a combination of mouth-wateringly sweet peach flavors, deliciously savory walnut pesto and dusted with parmesan cheese, it's a side-dish, starter or gourmet snack to remember!

Makes: 24 (serves 4-6)
Time: 35 mins
- Calories: 466
- Net carbs: 57g
- Protein: 10g
- Fat: 24g

Ingredients:
For the walnut pesto...
- 1/4 cup chopped walnuts
- 1 garlic clove, chopped
- 1-1/2 cups fresh arugula
- 1/4 cup extra-virgin olive oil
- Salt and pepper, to taste

For the bruschetta...
- 1 tablespoon olive oil plus additional for brushing bread, divided
- 1 large red onion, thinly sliced
- 1 teaspoon minced fresh rosemary
- 24 slices French bread baguette (3/8" thick)
- 2 garlic cloves, halved
- 2 small ripe peaches, cut into ¼" slices
- Shaved parmesan cheese
- Coarse salt

Method:
1. Grab the food processor and add the walnut and garlic. Hit the whizz button until finely chopped.
2. Add the arugula and whizz again.
3. Season well and add the oil whilst you keep whizzing.
4. Take a large skillet, pop over a medium heat and add a tablespoon of oil.
5. Add the onion and rosemary and cook for five minutes until soft.
6. Place the bread onto a flat surface and brush with remaining oil.
7. Pop under the grill or broiler until brown.
8. Remove and rub with garlic, spread with the pest and top with the fried onions, peaches and cheese.
9. Serve and enjoy.

Goat Cheese Mushrooms

Sometimes it's the simplest of the dishes that taste the best. With sweet roasted peppers, creamy goats' cheese and tender mushrooms, this one makes your heart sing and your taste buds beg for more.

Makes: 24 (serves 2)
Time: 30 mins

- Calories: 174
- Net carbs: 12g
- Protein: 10g
- Fat: 11g

Ingredients:

- 24 baby portobello mushrooms, stems removed
- 1/2 cup crumbled goat cheese
- 1/2 cup chopped drained roasted sweet red peppers
- Pepper, to taste
- 4 teaspoons olive oil
- Chopped fresh parsley

Method:

1. Preheat the oven to 375°F and grease a 15"10" baking sheet.
2. Place the mushrooms onto the baking sheet and top with 1 teaspoon of the cheese and 1 teaspoon of the red pepper.
3. Drizzle with oil and season well then cook for 15-18 minutes until tender.
4. Serve and enjoy.

Mediterranean Crab Phyllo Cups

These delightful crab snacks are perfect when you want to spoil yourself whilst keeping a check on your waistline. To be authentic, use the phyllo pastry, or substitute with slices of wholegrain bread.

Makes: 30
Time: 20 mins
- Calories: 34
- Net carbs: 3g
- Protein: 1g
- Fat: 2g

Ingredients:
- 1/2 cup cream cheese
- 1/2 teaspoon seafood seasoning
- 3/4 cup lump crabmeat, drained
- 2 x 1.9 oz. packages frozen miniature phyllo tart shells

To serve...
- Piri-Piri sauce or dried chili flakes

Method:
1. Take a small bowl and add the cream cheese and seasoning. Stir well.
2. Add the crab then stir again.
3. Divide the crab mixture into the tart shell, top with Piri-Piri sauce then serve and enjoy.

Dips & Spreads

Greek Eggplant Dip

Roasted eggplant, olive oil, garlic...Drool!!

Makes: 1 cup
Time: 1 hour 10 mins
- Calories: 97
- Net carbs: 16g
- Protein: 2g
- Fat: 2g

Ingredients:
- 1 lb. eggplant
- 1 red bell pepper
- 1 garlic clove, minced
- 1 ½ tablespoon olive oil
- 1 tablespoon red wine vinegar
- ¼ teaspoon salt
- 1 handful of parsley, chopped

Method:
1. Preheat oven to 400°F and grease a baking sheet.
2. Poke the eggplant with a fork and place onto the pan.
3. Pop into the oven for an hour until soft.
4. Remove from the oven and leave to cool.
5. Slice the eggplant then scoop out the insides, placing the flesh into your food processor.
6. Add the remaining ingredients and hit that whizz button until smooth.
7. Pop into the fridge to allow the flavors to blend then serve and enjoy.

Greek Parsley-Garlic Dip

You won't believe it when you try it, but there's no dairy whatsoever in this creamy and addictive dip.

Serves: 8
Time: 10 mins
- Calories: 250
- Net carbs: 3g
- Protein: 1g
- Fat: 25g

Ingredients:
- 1 ½ cup parsley leaves
- ½ onion
- 1 clove garlic
- 1 teaspoon capers
- ¼- ½ cup olive oil
- Juice from half a lemon
- 1-2 tablespoon red wine vinegar
- 1 cup stale bread
- Salt and pepper, to taste

Method:
1. Grab your food processor and add the parsley, onion, garlic and capers. Hit that whizz button until it becomes smooth.
2. Pop the bread into a bowl, moisten with a small amount of water then squeeze out all the liquid.
3. Add the bread to the parsley mixture and hit that whizz button again.
4. Keep the motor running whilst you slowly add the olive oil.
5. Add the vinegar, lemon juice and seasoning then stir well to combine.
6. Pop into the fridge to allow the flavors to blend.
7. Serve and enjoy.

Easy Ful Medammes

This fava bean dip comes right form the Middle East and it's similar in taste and texture to hummus. Using canned beans and the power of your food processor, you can create it in just the blink of an eye and enjoy it with breadsticks, fresh rustic bread or even as a dip for your crunchy veggies.

Serves: 4
Time: 10 mins

- Calories: 127
- Net carbs: 18g
- Protein: 6g
- Fat: 4g

Ingredients:

- 1 can fava beans
- 2 cloves garlic, finely chopped
- 1/2 teaspoon lemon juice
- 1 tablespoon tahini
- Pinch of salt
- 3 tablespoons hot water
- 1 tablespoon olive oil
- Optional garnish: parsley, finely chopped

Method:

1. Place the fava beans into a pan with the canning liquid, garlic and lemon juice.
2. Pop over a medium heat and bring to a boil then remove from the heat.
3. Mash with a fork or a potato masher then pop back over the heat.
4. Add the tahini, salt, water and olive oil and stir well to combine.
5. Serve and enjoy.

Red Pepper Dip with Feta Cheese and Greek Yogurt

Vibrant and creamy, this dip is a taste of the Mediterranean with about as many health benefits as you can manage to squeeze in. Delicious!

Serves: 4
Time: 5 mins
- Calories: 170
- Net carbs: 7g
- Protein: 7g
- Fat: 13g

Ingredients:
- 2 red peppers, roasted
- ¼ cup feta cheese, crumbled
- 2 tablespoons walnuts
- 3-4 tablespoons yogurt
- 1 tablespoon olive oil
- A pinch of oregano
- Pepper, to taste
- 1 clove garlic, minced

Method:
1. Grab your food processor and add all the ingredients.
2. Hit that whizz button until blended.
3. Transfer to a small bowl and pop into the fridge until ready to serve.

Tzatziki

Tzatziki is one of those dips that works brilliantly with just about any kind of Mediterranean dish. It keeps perfectly in your fridge for days, it's refreshing and delicious and it's far too moreish!

Makes: 1 cup
Time: 15 mins
- Calories: 53
- Net carbs: 4g
- Protein: 4g
- Fat: 5g

Ingredients:
- 1 medium cucumber, grated
- 1/2 cup plain Greek yogurt
- 1 tablespoon extra-virgin olive oil
- 2 teaspoons chopped fresh mint
- 1 1/2 teaspoons lemon juice
- 1 medium clove garlic, minced
- 1/4 teaspoon fine sea salt

Method:
1. Using your hands, squeeze the excess moisture from the cucumber and place into a small bowl.
2. Add the remaining ingredients, stir well then serve and enjoy.

Desserts & Sweet Treats

Greek Yogurt Chocolate Mousse

Yes, even chocolate mousse can be healthy when you do it Mediterranean style. Using honey, dark chocolate and a ton of love, you can create an indulgent desert that even the kids will love.

Serves: 4
Time: 2 hours

- Calories: 236
- Net carbs: 25g
- Protein: 15g
- Fat: 18g

Ingredients:

- 3/4 cup milk
- 3 ½ oz. dark chocolate
- 2 cups Greek yogurt
- 1 tablespoon honey or maple syrup
- 1/2 teaspoon vanilla extract

Method:

1. Grab a saucepan and add the chocolate and milk.
2. Place over a medium heat and stir until the chocolate melts.
3. Add the honey and vanilla and stir again until combined.
4. Pour into a bowl and add the yoghurt, then stir until combined.
5. Pop into the fridge for 2 hours then serve and enjoy.

Pistachio Mascarpone Cake with Roasted Figs

Even cakes can be (relatively) healthy when you approach it from a Mediterranean diet perspective. Of course, this awesome cake is still heavy on the calories so go easy on your portion sizes.

Serves: 9
Time: 45 mins
- Calories: 596
- Net carbs: 72g
- Protein: 8g
- Fat: 8g

Ingredients:
For the cake...
- 1 ½ oz. pistachios
- 2 ½ oz. powdered sugar
- 1 ½ oz. blanched almonds
- 2 whole eggs, whites and yolks separated
- 1 whole free-range egg
- ½ teaspoon cream of tartar
- 3 tablespoons + 1/2 cup sugar
- 2 oz. all-purpose flour

For the frosting...
- 1 cup heavy cream
- 8 oz. mascarpone cheese
- 1/2 cup powdered sugar

For the roasted figs...
- 12 ripe figs
- 1 tablespoon unsalted butter
- 2 tablespoons honey

Method:
1. Preheat your oven to 425°F and grease and line two 8" x 8" tins. Pop to one side.
2. Grab your food processor and add the pistachios, sugar and almonds. Hit whizz until the nuts are finely ground.
3. Transfer to a large bowl and add the eggs and egg yolks. Stir until combined.
4. Take another bowl and add the egg whites, cream of tartar, and 2 tablespoons of the sugar for the cake. Whisk until it forms stiff peaks.
5. Add the flour to the nut mixture and stir well. Then add the eggs and fold in.
6. Pour the batter into the two pans then bake for 10 minutes until the tops are golden.
7. Remove from the oven, remove from the tins and leave to cool.
8. Find an ovenproof dish and add the figs, butter and honey. Pop into the oven (still on 425°F) and cook for 10-15 minutes until bubbling. Leave to cool for a few minutes.

9. Meanwhile, place the remaining sugar and water into a saucepan and bring to the boil, stirring often to let the sugar dissolve. Remove from the heat and leave to cool.
10. Place the cream, mascarpone and sugar into a bowl and whisk until it forms peaks.
11. Place one of the cakes onto a plate and brush with sugar syrup. Add the frosting then top with the other cake.
12. Brush the syrup over the top and coat with the frosting. Pop into the fridge for an hour.
13. Decorate with the figs then serve and enjoy.

Vegan Coffee Tiramisu

Now THIS is a dish you should go make right now. I'm serious. It's about as healthy as a desert can possibly get, it's vegan and it's packed full of healthy iron, magnesium, proteins and a ton of other nutrients. Do you need any more excuses?

Serves: 8
Time: 30 mins
- Calories: 852
- Net carbs: 78g
- Protein: 13g
- Fat: 41g

Ingredients

For the base...
- ½ cup hazelnuts
- 1 cup almonds
- 7 Medjool dates
- 1 tablespoon coffee powder
- 2 tablespoons cacao powder
- 1 teaspoon vanilla extract
- Pinch of fine sea salt

For mousse layer...
- 1½ cup cashews, soaked overnight
- ¾ cup Medjool dates
- ⅓ cup melted raw dark chocolate
- ¼ cup maple syrup
- ⅔ cup almond milk, room temperature
- 4 tablespoons cacao butter, melted
- ⅓ cup cacao powder
- 2 teaspoon coffee powder

For the cream layer...
- ½ cup cashews, soaked overnight
- ⅔ cup cream
- 3 tablespoons coconut oil
- 2 tablespoons agave syrup
- 1 teaspoon vanilla extract

To serve...
- Cacao powder

Method:
1. Line a rectangular pan and pop to one side.
2. Grab your food processor and place the base ingredients inside. Hit that whizz button until the mixture goes crumbly and slightly sticky.
3. Press the mixture into the bottom of the pan and press down with a spatula. Pop into the freezer to firm up.

4. Get back to your food processor and add the mousse ingredients. Hit whizz until well combined and smooth.
5. Remove the pan from the freezer and pour the mousse over the top. Pop back into the freezer until firm.
6. Take your food processor again and add the ingredients for the cream layer. Whizz until smooth.
7. Remove the pan from the freezer when the mousse layer is firm and add the cream.
8. Pop back into the freezer and leave for 2 hours.
9. Sprinkle with the cacao powder and decorate with fresh fruit then serve and enjoy.

Mediterranean Pistachio No Bake Snack Bars

These easy snack bars make a nutritious and easy breakfast when you're on the run, a perfect post-workout nibble or a healthy treat when you really deserve something yummy.

Serves: 8
Time: 30 mins
- Calories: 220
- Net carbs: 20g
- Protein: 6g
- Fat: 12g

Ingredients:
- 20 pitted dates
- 1 1/4 cups roasted and salted pistachios
- 1 cup rolled old fashioned oats
- 2 tablespoons pistachio butter
- 1/4 cup unsweetened applesauce
- 1 teaspoon vanilla extract

Method:
1. Line an 8" x 8" with parchment paper and pop to one side.
2. Grab a food processor and add the dates. Hit that whizz button for 30 seconds until it forms a puree.
3. Add the pistachios and oats and pulse until crumbly.
4. Add the pistachio butter, applesauce and vanilla and pulse again until it forms a dough.
5. Transfer to your pre-prepared tin and press down with a spatula.
6. Pop into the fridge until firm.
7. Serve and enjoy!

Final words

Hey! Welcome to the end of the book. It's great to have you here still!

As you've followed me through the pages of this short book, you should have felt that jolt of inspiration rush through your veins, felt your mouth start to water in anticipation and experienced a strange urge to run into the kitchen and get cooking.

Don't worry- you're not going mad! That's exactly the effect that the Mediterranean diet has on me too.

Because, as you've seen, it's not only utterly delicious, packed with an astonishing array of antioxidants, phytonutrients, vitamins and minerals and perfect for keeping your waistline in shape, it's also awesome for your health and looks vibrant and inspiring.

Whether you've come to the Mediterranean diet to lose weight, to move towards a more plant-based diet or you're getting some health issues in check, I can guarantee you'll find the solution in the pages of this book.

So, what's stopping you? Choose your favorite recipe in this book, make yourself a grocery list then head out to buy the ingredients for the first meal of the rest of your life.

And finally, if you've loved reading this book and want to help me spread the word about this fabulous diet, please take a second to head over to Amazon and leave me a quick review! Even a word or two would make a massive difference to me.

Thank you and happy cooking!

Made in the USA
Middletown, DE
27 September 2019